The Wonder of What We Eat

How Our Incredible Food,
Our Incredible Bodies,
And Our Incredible Planet
Are Connected

Ritu Saluja-Sharma MD

Disclaimer

The content of this book is for general informational purposes only. Each person's physical, emotional, and spiritual condition is unique. The instruction in this book is not meant to be used, nor should it be used, to diagnose or treat any medical condition or to replace the services of your physician or other healthcare provider. The advice and strategies contained in the book may not be suitable for all readers. Neither the author, publisher, nor any of their employees or representatives guarantees the accuracy of information in this book or its usefulness to a particular reader, nor are they responsible for any damage or negative consequence that may result from any treatment, action taken, or inaction by any person reading or following the information in this book.

Copyright © 2025 Ritu Saluja-Sharma
Head Heart Hands LLC, Gaithersburg, MD
headhearthandsmd.com
Illustrator: Navdeep Kaur Komal
ISBN: 979-8-9990505-1-9

All rights reserved. No part of this publication may be reproduced, distributed, or transmitted in any form or by any means, including photocopying, recording or other electronic or mechanical methods, without the prior written permission of the publisher. For permissions, contact headhearthandsmd@gmail.com.

DEDICATION

To the parents who are doing their best to nourish their children in a world that doesn't make it easy.

To the teachers who plant seeds of knowledge that grow into lifelong habits.

And most of all, to the kids—may you always stay curious about your bodies, your food, and the power you hold to shape your future.

CONTENTS

Preface to Parents.. i
Introduction... iv

Part 1: Our Bodies Are Extraordinary
1. Our Incredible Digestive Tract............................ 2

Part 2: Our Food Is Extraordinary
2. Our Food is Energy... 8
3. Our Food is the Building Blocks of Our Bodies.... 17
4. Our Food is Micronutrients.................................. 24
5. Our Food is Food for our Gut Microbiome............ 36
6. Our Food is Instructions & Information................. 44

Part 3: Our Earth Is Extraordinary
7. Choosing Extraordinary Food.............................. 60
8. Creating an Incredible Plate................................. 76

Part 4: The Connection Between Our Bodies, Our Food, And Our Earth Is Extraordinary
9. Our Food and Our Farms..................................... 86
10. Our Incredible Food, Our Incredible Bodies, Our Incredible Earth... 101

Afterword... 111
Glossary... 112
About the Author.. 120
Acknowledgements.. 122

PREFACE TO PARENTS

In a world where ultra-processed food dominates kids' diets and the childhood obesity epidemic is soaring, our food system and diet culture are failing our children.

Our system is failing adults too.

Six out of 10 adults in the U.S. have a chronic disease. Four out of 10 have two or more chronic diseases. In the U.S., we spend more money on healthcare than any other nation, but we have among the highest rates of chronic disease in the world.

As an emergency physician who has worked on the front lines of our healthcare system for almost twenty years, every day I see patients suffering with conditions that could likely have been prevented and can potentially still be reversed. Yet most patients don't get the help they need to prevent or reverse disease.

While searching for answers and a better solution, I continued my training and earned a second board certification in Lifestyle Medicine. Lifestyle Medicine focuses on helping people prevent and reverse our most common diseases by targeting the root causes of their problems.

Over the past five years, I have been working with adults to help them understand the power of food, understand the power of their bodies, and help them make positive changes to their diet and lifestyle in order to transform their health. The results have been extraordinary. When provided this help, adults have lowered their blood sugars, blood pressure, and cholesterol, lost weight, increased their energy, decreased their pain, and improved their quality of life. Many have even reduced or eliminated their need for medications.

Yet, as exciting as it is for adults to transform their health, many are left asking, why didn't I get this help sooner? Why didn't I learn about food and nutrition when I was a kid?

I had these same questions. I only discovered the power of food after studying Lifestyle Medicine, after navigating my own health journey. This was after decades of schooling that taught me surprisingly little about food.

I wrote this book to empower kids with the essential nutrition education that most adults don't even know- and worse, don't know where to find. Learning this information as kids can change the trajectory of their health and the trajectory of their life.

But just nutrition education and knowledge are not enough. In order to help adults and kids make meaningful change, a healthy mindset about food and their body is essential.

In our toxic diet culture, which emphasizes numbers on a scale and numbers of calories, food is often viewed as the enemy. We learn that when we eat food, we must burn it off by exercising. We learn that in order to be healthy, we need to use our willpower and eat less to lose weight. These unhealthy messages set us up to develop an unhealthy relationship with food, and an unhealthy relationship with our body.

This book explores the incredible power of food and the extraordinary power of the human body. It helps kids look at food as more than just calories, and their bodies/health as more than just numbers on a scale. Understanding these simple, yet revolutionary concepts can be life changing (even for adults). By teaching kids about food and health in this way, it can shape their mindset and their choices for their entire life.

In addition to being a book that kids can read themselves at home, this book was also designed to be incorporated into school curriculums. To effectively combat our epidemics of chronic disease and obesity, we must empower kids of all demographics with essential nutrition knowledge and provide a positive foundation for how they think about food and their body.

I am excited to be working with school systems to incorporate these concepts into their curriculum, and also to be providing input to change the health curriculum standards on the state level.

I encourage you to read this book together with your kids. There's also a workbook you can use to practice what you learn, and a corresponding cookbook filled with delicious, healthy recipes to try at home.

Together, let's build a healthier, happier future—one plate, one choice, and one kid at a time.

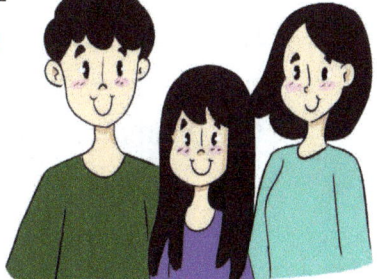

INTRODUCTION

Have you ever thought about how much time you spend eating every single day? Over the course of your life, how much time will you spend just eating? The answer is A LOT!

Everyone is different, but most people around the world spend more than 67 minutes a day just eating. This adds up to more than 32,000 hours, or eating day and night without stopping for almost 4 years.

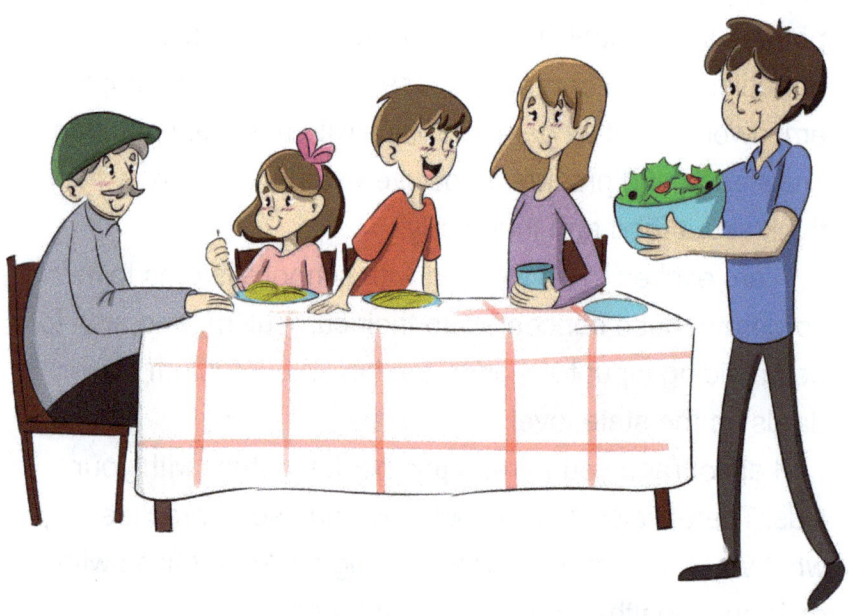

So eating is an enormous part of our life! And this is for good reason. Food is super important! Humans cannot survive without food. It's extraordinarily powerful. Food has an immediate effect on the way your body feels, and it

also determines the health of your body in the future.
And the food you eat is not just connected to the health of your body, it is also connected to the health of our planet.

How can something as ordinary as food be so powerful?

The truth of the matter is that most adults don't even know the answer to this question.

Most adults were never taught much about food, and they don't recognize the power of food. But if they did, our world would be very different. Adults would be healthier. Kids would be healthier. Our Earth would be healthier too.

For many adults, they have mostly just learned that when they eat too much, they gain weight. Some adults have learned that to improve their health they need to lose weight by eating less food.

But thinking about food and the health of your body in this way is too simple! Not only that, when we think about food and our health in this way, we aren't appreciating how incredible our food is, and how incredible our bodies are.

Personally, I wasn't taught anything about food for most of my life— not in school, not in college, not in medical school, and not even when I was training to be an Emergency Room doctor. For most of my life, I thought I knew a lot about food— but I didn't know how much I didn't know!

Even though I am a doctor, there were a lot of

times that I didn't feel well, and I didn't know why. For example, when I was a kid, I had lots of stomachaches, which were pretty miserable. The stomachaches continued even when I was an adult. I never knew what to do about it, and I always thought there was something wrong with my body. But when I started learning more about how food and my body are connected, I was able to make changes to what I was eating. Now I feel so much better, and those stomachaches are gone! It makes me sad that I suffered for so many years unnecessarily and felt bad about my body because I was never taught about food.

Now as a doctor, I help my patients improve their health using the power of food. Our bodies are extraordinary, and when we harness the power of food, our bodies are often capable of healing themselves. But here's something even more amazing— the same food that makes us stronger and healthier can also make our Earth healthier too.

How is it that our food, our bodies, and our planet are so interconnected? Why does what we eat matter so much?

In order to understand this extraordinary connection, we must understand food, understand how our bodies use our food, and understand where our food comes from.

Are you ready to learn more?

PART 1:
OUR BODIES ARE **EXTRAORDINARY**

CHAPTER 1
OUR INCREDIBLE DIGESTIVE TRACT

Have you ever wondered what happens to your food when you eat? Or how the food you eat becomes waste (poop)? How does it get from your mouth to the other end? What happens in between?

The first step to understanding the extraordinary power of food is to explore what happens when you eat. Where does your food go?

Imagine you are hungry, and you eat lunch. Every bite of food you eat goes on an amazing journey through your digestive system! The first stop is your mouth. As soon as you take a bite of food, your mouth starts working on it. You use your teeth to take bites of food and then to chew it into little pieces. Your tongue helps you move your food around your mouth and allows you to taste your food. The salivary glands in your mouth make saliva (also called spit) that is a watery liquid that contains <u>enzymes</u> (chemicals) that start to break down your food. The saliva also makes your food easier to swallow.

When you swallow, food is pushed down your esophagus, which is a tube that leads from your throat to your stomach. Your stomach is filled with acid that helps to break down your food even more. By the time your food leaves your stomach, it has become a thick liquid called <u>chyme</u>.

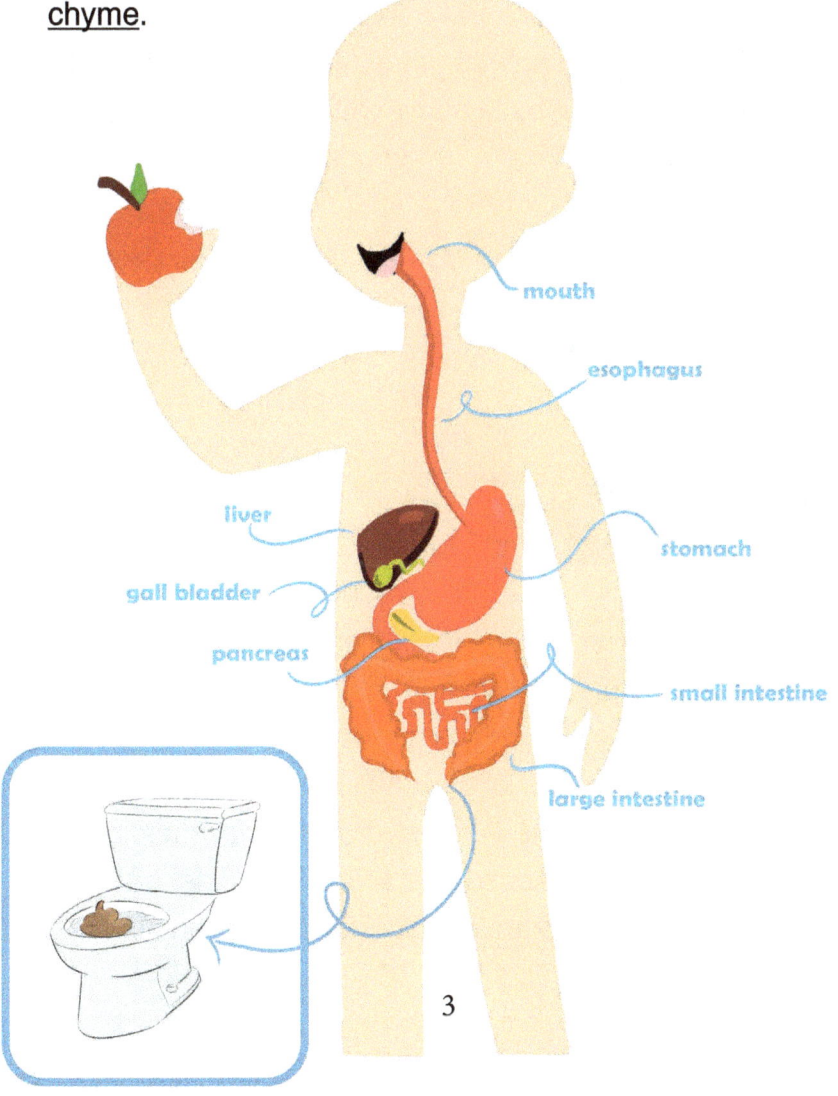

Have you ever eaten too much and had a stomachache? When you eat a big meal, your stomach can actually stretch to hold all the food, and this will cause you to feel really full.

The next step after your stomach is your small intestine, which is a long, winding, narrow tube, where most of the work of digesting your food happens. The small intestine tube is about the width of your index finger, but it is not small at all! It is actually very long.

Can you guess the length of the small intestine? It is hard to believe, but by the time you are 10 years old, your small intestine is about 16 feet long. (That's about the height of a giraffe). By the time you're an adult, your small intestine could be about 20 feet long!! (That's about the length of a small school bus!)

Not only that, but the inner lining of the small intestine is also impressively large. The small intestine tube has millions of villi, which are microscopic fingerlike projections that create more surface area to absorb the nutrients from your food. If you stretch out the inner lining of the small intestine, so that all the villi, folds, and scrunched up sections are flat, your small intestine inner lining would be bigger than the inside of a school bus!

After you eat, it typically takes about 6-8 hours for food to move through your stomach and small intestine. After that, it goes to your large intestine, also known as your colon. Once your food gets to your large intestine, most of the work of absorbing the nutrients is finished. The main job of the large intestine is to remove water from what is left, so that it becomes more compact. All that is left is solid waste (poop), which you get rid of when you go to the bathroom.

Our bodies are incredible!! There is so much going on from our head down to our toes and every place in between! But believe it or not, this is just the beginning of what happens to your food!

After your food is absorbed from your small intestine, it goes on an even more amazing journey through your body. Your food plays a role in everything your body does, from giving you energy to determining your future.

Are you ready to learn more about this extraordinary connection? Let's get started!

PART 2:
OUR FOOD IS **EXTRAORDINARY**

CHAPTER 2
OUR FOOD IS ENERGY

Have you ever felt tired in the afternoon after lunch? Maybe like you want to take a nap? Or have you ever felt lazy and "blah" in the morning and wished that you had more energy?

The food you eat determines your energy level.

To drive a car, it needs fuel or electricity to function. In the same way, your body needs fuel to function. Where does our fuel or energy come from? It comes from the food we eat.

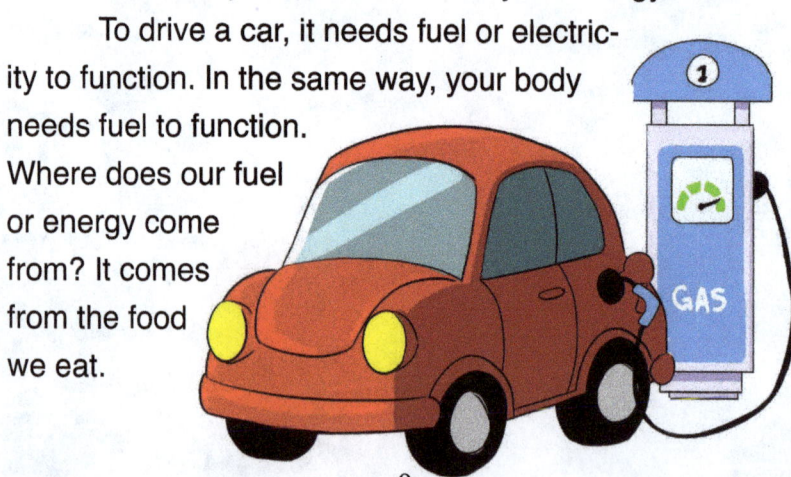

Food contains nutrients, and nutrients can be divided into 2 categories: macronutrients and micronutrients.

"Macro" means large. Macronutrients are called this because these are the nutrients that your body needs in large amounts to provide your body with energy and to keep you healthy. The three main macronutrients are:
1. Carbohydrates
2. Proteins
3. Fats

Carbohydrates are your body's preferred source of energy. Carbohydrates include foods like fruits, vegetables, beans, lentils, rice, bread, pasta, crackers, and so much more.

When you eat carbohydrates, your body breaks them down into simple sugars, which are the sugars that your body can absorb and use for energy. Glucose is a simple sugar which is your primary source of energy, allowing all your cells to function. If you hear someone talk about their glucose level, they're talking about the sugar in their blood. Your blood sugar is the glucose in your blood that circulates to all your cells to give them what they need to function- what they need to make energy.

Do you know what part of your body uses the most glucose?

Believe it or not, it's your brain. Your brain is amazing! It is constantly working and controlling almost everything that is happening in your body by sending messages through your nerve cells. Your nerve cells act like tiny telephone wires, and the messages they transmit instruct your cells what to do. Because your brain is rich in nerve cells, it demands the most energy.

But it's not just your brain that needs glucose. All your cells need glucose to function. Think of glucose as the fuel that powers each and every one your cells to do everything they need to do.

So, if glucose is so important for your energy, and glucose mostly comes from carbohydrates, this makes carbohydrates super important.

But not all carbohydrates are the same, and the type of carbohydrates that you eat has a big impact on your energy level. There are two types of carbohydrates: <u>simple carbohydrates</u>, and <u>complex carbohydrates</u>.

Simple carbohydrates are made of simple sugars. This type of carbohydrate can be digested and absorbed very quickly. When you eat simple carbohydrates, your blood sugar increases fast. Examples of simple carbohydrates are sugar, candy, sweet drinks (including soda and fruit juice), most crackers and cookies and white bread.

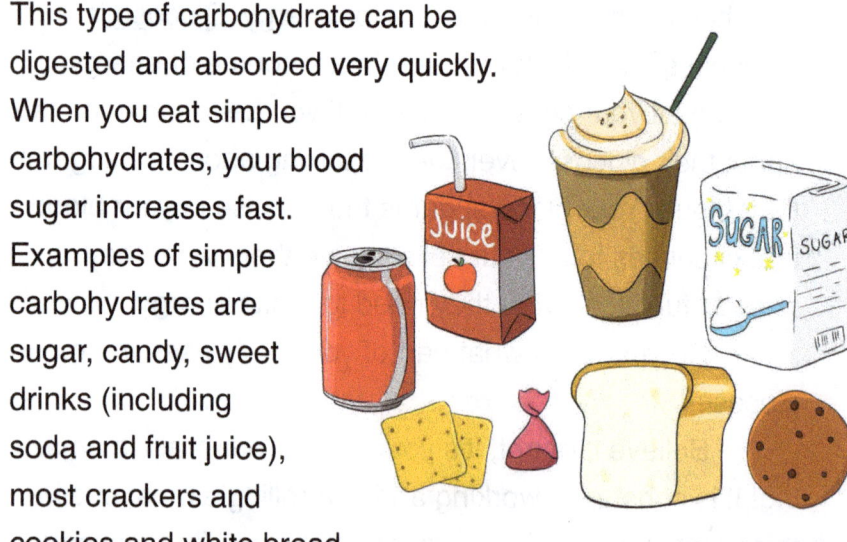

When you eat these simple carbohydrates, the simple sugars can be absorbed very quickly. This can give you a burst of energy when your blood sugar increases quickly, but then after your food is quickly digested and absorbed, your blood sugar can drop really fast too. For this reason, when you eat simple carbohydrates, you will feel energy for a bit, but then soon after, your energy level may drop, and you may feel tired or sluggish.

The other type of carbohydrate is called complex. **Complex carbohydrates** need to be broken down into simple sugars before your body can absorb them. The process of breaking down complex carbohydrates takes your body time. Because of that, the energy they give you can be sustained good energy that lasts all day long. Fruits, vegetables, <u>whole grains</u>, beans, and lentils are all complex carbohydrates.

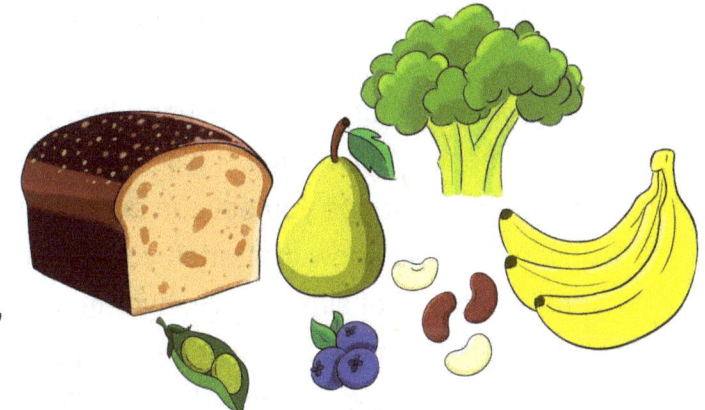

As opposed to simple carbohydrates, that are often made in factories, complex carbohydrates are mostly found in nature. Complex carbohydrates are the carbohydrates that nature designed for us to eat. Complex carbohydrates take longer for our stomach and small intestine to digest because they are naturally packaged with a nutrient called <u>fiber</u>. As our body slowly breaks down the carbohydrates packaged with fiber, glucose is gradually absorbed into our blood stream, our energy levels will go up, and they won't quickly drop like when you eat simple carbohydrates. For this reason, complex carbohydrates will give us good, lasting energy, without the energy crashes that we get when we eat simple carbohydrates.

This is why professional athletes who want to improve their energy level, performance, and endurance (how long they can play) eat mostly complex carbohydrates rather than simple carbohydrates. Meals rich in whole grains, fruits and vegetables, beans and lentils are excellent choices for athletes, to give them energy that lasts.

Not only that, but considering that your brain is the biggest user of your energy, it also makes sense that the type of carbohydrates you eat can even impact your brain function. Did you know that when you eat complex carbohydrates instead of simple carbohydrates, and your blood sugar levels are more stable, it also helps your brain? Eating more complex carbohydrates instead of simple carbohydrates can have a positive effect on your mood, your concentration, and your memory. This means eating more complex carbohydrates can help you do better in school, perform better in sports, and feel happier too!

What Is A Whole Grain Versus A Refined Grain?

Whole grains are complex carbohydrates and refined grains are simple carbohydrates. What is the difference?

A whole grain consists of three parts: The bran, germ, and the endosperm.

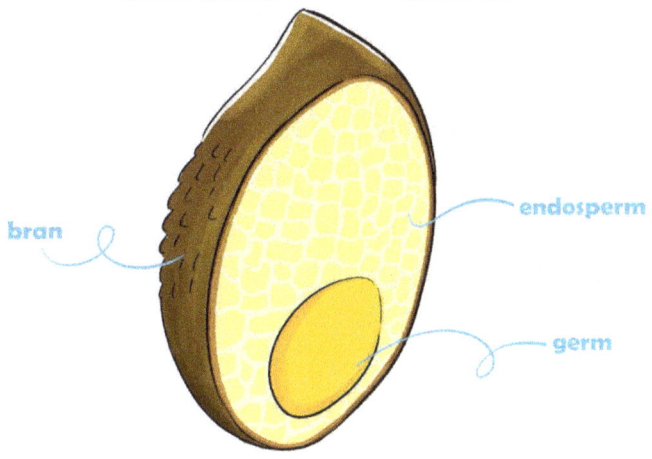

Bran:	The bran is the outer skin of the edible kernel. It contains important antioxidants, B vitamins and fiber.
Germ:	The germ is the embryo which has the potential to sprout into a new plant. It contains many B vitamins, some protein, minerals, and healthy fats.
Endo-sperm:	The endosperm is the germ's food supply, so it can grow roots and sprout. The endosperm is the largest part, and contains starchy carbohydrates, protein, and small amounts of vitamins and minerals. Gluten is found in the endosperm.

All grains start as whole grains, which are the entire seed of the plant with all three parts.

Refined grain is the term used to refer to grains that are not whole, because they are missing one or more of their three key parts (bran, germ, or endosperm). White flour and white rice are refined grains, for instance, because both have had their bran and germ removed, leaving only the endosperm.

Refining a grain removes the fiber, some of the protein content from the grain, and many of the nutrients. For this reason, when you eat refined grains, the effect is similar to when you are eating candy or sugar— your blood sugar goes up really quickly because there is no fiber.

Examples of refined grains are white rice, white bread, and most cookies, crackers, and snack foods that are found in packages.

A better choice is to eat whole grains like brown rice, <u>quinoa</u>, or 100% whole grain bread, which are complex carbohydrates, and will give you lasting, good energy.

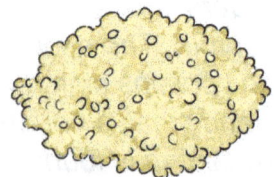
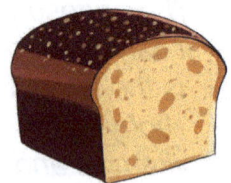

So how can you tell if you are eating simple carbohydrates or complex carbohydrates? Unfortunately, most adults don't even know the answer to this question. This is because most adults were never taught about nutrition when they were kids! Lucky for you, you will know better!

Often when adults look at food labels, they just look at the number of calories. Calories are a measure of the amount of energy that is in food.

But the number of calories in food does not tell us whether we are eating simple carbohydrates or complex carbohydrates. It doesn't tell us if we are going to get lasting sustained energy from the food, or whether the food will lead to an energy burst and then energy crash. Calories are only a measure of the amount of energy in food. For this reason, just looking at calories is very misleading.

Consider this, you just came home from school, and you are having a snack before soccer practice. You could choose a banana which is about 105 calories, or a package of Goldfish crackers, which is 200 calories. Which snack do you think is going to give you more energy for your soccer practice? Which snack would you choose?

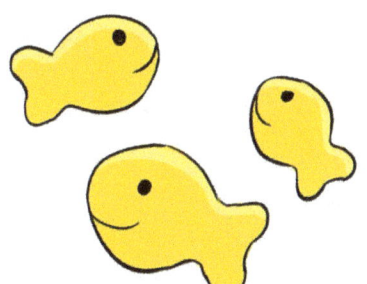
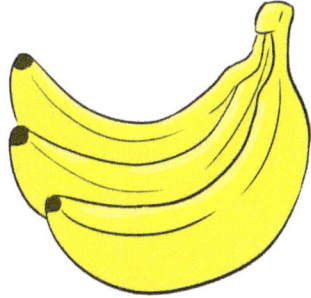

If you just rely on the number of calories, you may choose the Goldfish, but the banana will give you more sustained energy! The banana is a complex carbohydrate with fiber and lots of nutrients. When you eat it, your body will slowly digest it, to give you more lasting energy. In contrast, when you eat the Goldfish crackers, which are made in a factory, the food manufacturers have stripped most of the fiber and nutrients from the wheat, and your body can quickly break them down. You may get a quick rush of energy, but this probably won't even last long enough for you to get to your soccer practice. The banana is a much better choice!

So next time you want a snack, what kind of snack will you choose?

Rather than counting calories, a better approach is to focus on eating foods that will give you lasting, sustained energy. Here are some suggestions:

- Fruits: apples, pears, berries
- Avocado on whole grain toast
- Nuts
- Cheese and whole grain crackers
- Banana and peanut butter

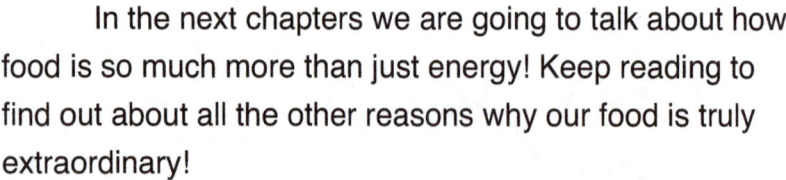

In the next chapters we are going to talk about how food is so much more than just energy! Keep reading to find out about all the other reasons why our food is truly extraordinary!

CHAPTER 3
OUR FOOD IS THE BUILDING BLOCKS OF OUR BODIES

Have you ever wondered what your body is made of? The human body is made up of trillions of tiny cells!

Cells are the tiny building blocks that make up all living things, including plants, animals, and humans! There are lots of different kinds of cells in your body, and they are too small to see without a microscope. Each cell contains your DNA, which is like a set of instructions that tells your cells what to become and what to do.

These tiny cells then stack tightly together to make tissue, the material that makes living things. All your organs (like your heart, your brain, your skin, and your muscles) are made up of tissue.

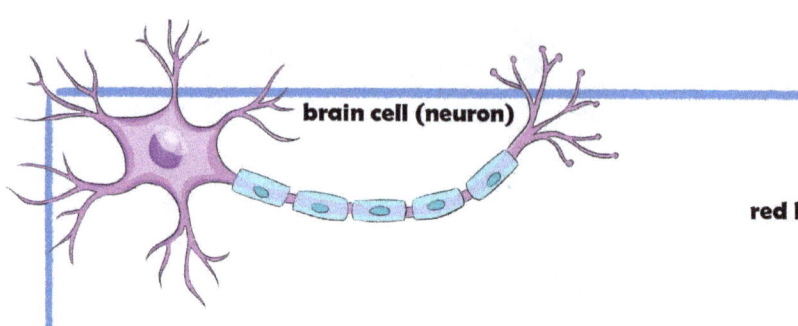
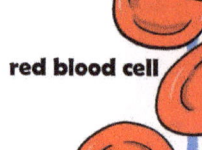

What Are Cells?

Depending on what they do, cells come in all shapes and sizes. Your skin cells come together to form your skin that covers your body. Your brain is made of nerve cells called neurons, but there are also long nerve cells that carry messages from your brain to all around your body. Your blood is made of many different types of blood cells, including red blood cells that carry oxygen around your body to your cells. Your white blood cells are part of your immune system and help your body fight infections and heal when you get injured.

The food you eat is important for all of your cells to be able to function.

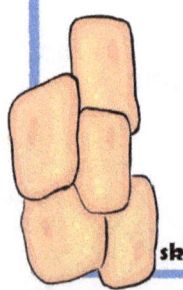

In the last chapter we learned that carbohydrates are your body's main source of energy. But there are two other macronutrients we didn't learn about yet— proteins and fats. When you eat proteins and fats, they can supply you energy too— but they are also important for other reasons! Proteins are the building blocks of our body and fats are an important component in all our cells.

So quite literally, we need proteins and fats to exist!

First let's talk about proteins. Your body contains large amounts of protein, because protein is the primary component of all cells. For example, your muscle cells, your skin cells, your bone cells, and your blood cells are all built mostly of protein.

Did you know that we have about 30 trillion cells in our body (4 times more than the number of grains of sand on Earth)? And did you know that every day your body replaces about 330 billion new cells? This means that every second you are replacing about 3.8 million cells!

For this reason, it is super important that you eat enough protein every day to grow, to build more cells, and to repair and replace your cells. This is especially important for growing kids like you!

So where do we find protein?

Protein can be found in foods that come from animals, like meat, dairy, and eggs, and protein is also in plants. Beans, lentils, peas, <u>edamame</u>, tofu, nuts, and even seeds all have a lot of protein.

Protein Makes Up The Building Blocks Of Our Muscles

Protein is important for everyone, but it's especially important if you're growing and active, because it helps you get stronger and build muscles.

Our muscle cells are made up of long strands of protein called <u>myofibrils</u>. To create these myofibrils and form muscle, we need to eat enough protein.

But it's not just protein that is important to build muscle. You also need to use your muscles to build muscle! Activities like playing on the monkey bars and climbing will help you build muscles and get stronger. Not only that, but playing sports, like soccer, running, and swimming, or dancing where you are using your muscles, will also help your muscles grow.

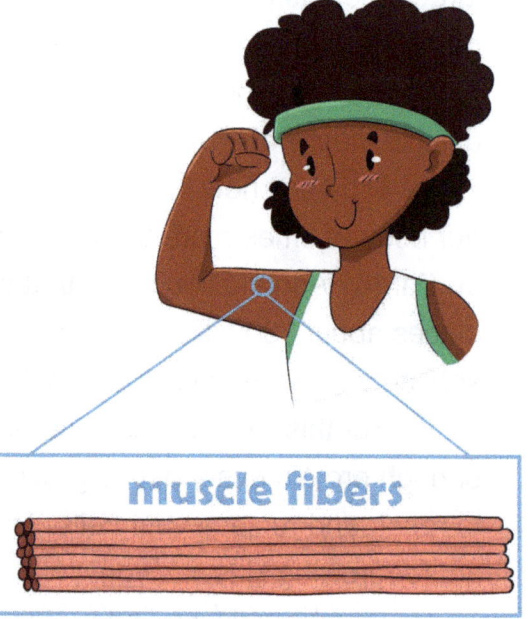
muscle fibers

What are your favorite activities where you are using your muscles and getting stronger?

Next let's talk about the third macronutrient: fats. Fats are needed for healthy cells. They are used to build the outer covering of our cells (our cell membranes). Fats also help our body absorb certain vitamins, including vitamin A, D, E, and K. They are also essential for building hormones, which act like messengers to guide how our body works.

Fats are also super important for our brain health! Did you know that our brain is made up of about 60% fat? Hard to believe, right? This is important, because the fat that we eat can have a big impact on our learning, our memory, and our mental processing, meaning how we put thoughts together.

Fat can be found in lots of food, including oil, butter, meat, dairy, nuts, nut butters, seeds, and avocados. There are lots of different kinds of fat, and the type of fat that we eat matters. The main types of fats are trans fats, saturated fats, monounsaturated fats, and <u>polyunsaturated fats</u>. Let's talk about each of them briefly.

Trans fats are the unhealthiest fats for our bodies. They are mostly human-made, created by changing the natural chemical structure of vegetable oils. Trans fats are mostly found in food that is made in factories, with lots of food processing to make them stay fresh tasting for longer. Thankfully trans fats have been mostly banned in the U.S.—which means that food companies in the U.S. are not allowed to add them to food anymore. But even though trans fats are banned, they may still be found in small amounts in packaged foods like microwave popcorn, refrigerated doughs (like biscuits and rolls), and packaged pre-made baked goods. Trans fats can also be found in fried foods.

Saturated fat is solid at room temperature, like the fat in butter or the fat you might find around the outside of a steak. It is often found in food from animals, like meat, cheese, and whole milk. You also find saturated fat in packaged baked goods that use saturated plant fats such as palm oil and coconut oil. Eating too much saturated fat can be unhealthy for your heart and blood vessels.

The monounsaturated fats are one of the healthiest fats! You can find this type of healthy fat in foods like olives, avocados, most nuts, and even nut butters (including peanut butter and almond butter). These fats are the types of fats that we want to aim to include in our diet! In fact, eating nuts every day (if you are not allergic) is one of the best things you can do for your health!

There are 2 types of polyunsaturated fats— omega-3 fatty acids and omega-6 fatty acids. Omega-3's and omega-6's sound similar, but there is actually a big difference between these types of fats. Our body can't make these fats, so we must get them from the food we eat.

Omega-3 fats are found in some types of fish (including salmon and tuna), walnuts, chia seeds, flax seeds, and hemp seeds. There has been a lot of research which shows that eating omega-3 fatty acids can be beneficial for our heart health and brain health!

When eaten in small amounts, omega-6 fats can also be good for your health. Unfortunately, though, most people eat way too much omega-6 fat. This is because omega-6 fats are found in the oils used to make most packaged food, fast food, and fried foods. If we are eating a lot of packaged foods, fast foods, and fried foods, and not a lot of fish, nuts, and seeds we may likely be getting too much of the omega-6 fats, and not enough of the omega-3's.

So, the bottom line is that not all fat is the same. Eat more olives, avocados, nuts, seeds, and fish as your sources of fat, rather than eating the fat in red meat, fast food, and packaged food made in factories. And since your brain is made mostly 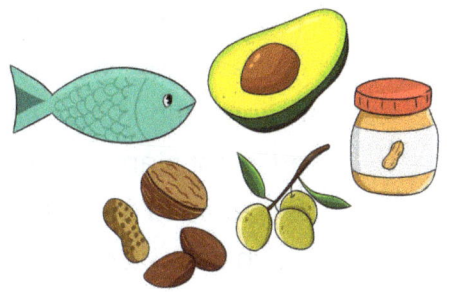 of fat, eating the healthy types of fat can make a big difference in your brain health! Eating healthy fat can even improve your ability to concentrate, to learn, and to remember things!

Healthy protein and healthy fats are incredible!

CHAPTER 4
OUR FOOD IS MICRONUTRIENTS

Every day, all day long, your body is doing amazing things. Your body is constantly making new cells. Your brain is constantly sending messages through your nerves to your entire body to control everything that you do. Your immune system is constantly working to protect you from infections and to heal you when you are injured. Your heart is constantly pumping, beating over 100,000 times a day, to send blood and oxygen all around your body through your blood vessels. Your body is amazing!!

In order to perform all of these tasks, and much, much more, you need some essential micronutrients. In the last two chapters we talked about the macronutrients-- carbohydrates, protein, and fat, which provide energy and are the building blocks of the body. Now we are going to talk about micronutrients, also called vitamins and minerals, which are the nutrients that your body needs in small amounts but cannot produce itself. Even though "micro" means tiny, micronutrients are super important and super powerful!

There are two main types of micronutrients: vitamins and minerals.

Vitamins are organic substances, which means they are made by plants or animals. Minerals, on the other hand, originally come from the soil or water, and are absorbed by plants or eaten by animals.

An example of a vitamin is Vitamin C, which is found in lots of fruits and vegetables including oranges, bell peppers, and strawberries. Vitamin C is needed for your body to create collagen, an important protein that strengthens your bones, skin, and blood vessels. In fact, there is more collagen in your body than any other protein! Vitamin C is also essential for your immune system to function properly, so that you can fight off germs and illnesses. Vitamin C also is needed to protect your cells from damage and to heal your wounds.

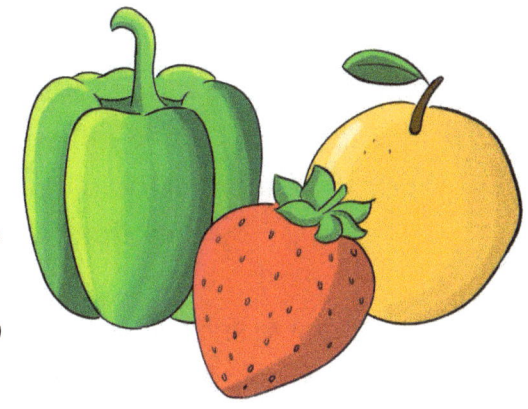

An example of a mineral is <u>magnesium</u>. Magnesium is found in green leafy vegetables (including spinach, kale, collards, and Swiss chard), nuts and seeds (like almonds, cashews, chia seeds and pumpkin seeds), and beans (including black beans and lima beans). Magnesium is needed for over 300 chemical reactions that happen in your body, so that your body can function properly. Magnesium is needed for your muscles to function, for 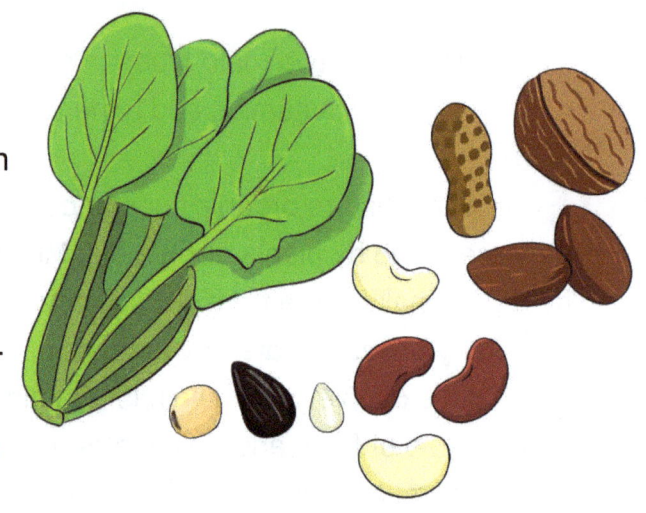 your nerves to carry messages from your brain to your body, for your heart to beat properly, for your immune system to function at its best, for your body to create strong bones and teeth, and for so much more!

When you are eating foods that are rich in micronutrients (vitamins and minerals), you are giving your body the essential tools it needs to be strong and to function at its best.

Want to know what else the micronutrients you eat are doing in your body? Take a look…

Did You Know That The Micronutrients In Your Food Can Affect Your Mood?

Believe it or not the micronutrients in your food can have a big impact on how happy or sad you feel. This is because many vitamins and minerals play a big role in how your brain works. When you eat foods that are rich in micronutrients, it can help you feel calmer, happier, and more focused. On the other hand, if you are not getting enough essential nutrients, it may have a negative impact on your mood, your anxiety levels, and your ability to concentrate.

Some of the nutrients that scientists believe may affect our mood include vitamin D (found in fatty fish and made when our bodies are exposed to the sun), the B vitamins (B6, B12, and B9 [folate] found in leafy greens, whole grains, meat, and beans), magnesium (found in beans, greens, nuts, and seeds), omega 3 fatty acids (found in fatty fish, walnuts, chia seeds, and flax seeds), and zinc (found in pumpkin seeds).

While more research is needed to prove exactly which nutrients impact our brain health and mood, and to what degree, we do know that eating a balanced diet with lots of micronutrients helps all of our organs function at their best, including our brain!

MICRONUTRIENT CHART

Nutrient	Function	Food Sources
Calcium	Builds strong bones and teeth and keeps your muscles moving.	Broccoli | Almonds | Tofu | Milk | Fortified soy milk
Iron	Helps your body make blood, which carries oxygen around your body to give you energy.	Spinach | Lentils | Meat | Fish | Tofu | Pumpkin Seeds
Magnesium	Helps muscles work, keeps bones strong, and supports energy production.	Green Leafy Vegetables | Pumpkin Seeds | Black Beans | Almonds
Potassium	Helps your muscles move and keeps your heart beating steadily.	Bananas | Sweet potatoes | Beans | Avocados
Vitamin A	Keeps your eyes sharp, helps you grow, and protects you from getting sick.	Carrots | Sweet potatoes | Spinach | Kale | Cantaloupe
Vitamin B1 (Thiamine)	Turns food into energy so you can run, jump, and play, and keeps your nerves healthy.	Whole grains | Beans | Nuts | Seeds
Vitamin B12 (Cobalamin)	Keeps your nerves and blood healthy and helps make your DNA.	Fish | Dairy Foods | Eggs
Vitamin B2 (Riboflavin)	Helps you get energy from food and keeps your skin and eyes strong.	Milk | Yogurt | Spinach | Mushrooms
Vitamin B3 (Niacin)	Helps your body break down food and use it for energy.	Peanuts | Mushrooms | Whole grains | Peas

MICRONUTRIENT CHART

Vitamin B5 (Pantothenic Acid)	Supports making energy and important hormones your body needs.	Avocados	Sweet potatoes	Broccoli	Whole grains
Vitamin B6 (Pyridoxine)	Helps your brain think clearly and makes important blood cells.	Bananas	Chickpeas	Spinach	Potatoes
Vitamin B7 (Biotin)	Helps your body use energy and keeps your skin, hair, and nails healthy.	Almonds	Sweet potatoes	Spinach	Eggs
Vitamin B9 (Folate)	Builds new cells to help you grow and heal faster.	Spinach	Broccoli	Lentils	Oranges
Vitamin C	Strengthens your immune system and helps your body heal cuts and bruises.	Oranges	Strawberries	Bell peppers	Broccoli
Vitamin D	Helps you absorb calcium to build strong bones and teeth. Helps your immune system and brain stay strong and healthy.	Sunlight	Mushrooms	Fish	Fortified Soy Milk	Fortified Dairy Products
Vitamin E	Protects your cells and keeps your skin and eyes healthy.	Almonds	Sunflower seeds	Spinach	Avocados
Vitamin K	Helps your blood clot if you get a cut and keeps your bones strong.	Broccoli	Spinach	Kale	Green beans
Zinc	Strengthens your immune system and helps heal wounds quickly.	Pumpkin Seeds	Cashews	Chickpeas	Lentils

In addition to vitamins and minerals that are essential, which means your body cannot produce them but needs them to function and stay alive, there is also another group of nutrients called <u>phytonutrients</u>. Phytonutrients are chemicals that are produced by plants which help your body function at its best. Scientists are still trying to identify all of these beneficial compounds in plants, and so far, there are more than 10,000 known phytonutrients! Amazingly, there are also probably a lot more phytonutrients that we have not yet recognized! These amazing chemicals in plants help to explain why eating fruits and vegetables is so beneficial for our bodies.

Here are some examples:

<u>Carotenoids</u> are a family of powerful phytonutrients, found in foods like carrots, sweet potatoes, and mangoes that give fruits and vegetables their bright red, yellow and orange colors. Carotenoids keep your eyes healthy and strong, protect your cells against damage, and boost your immune system.

<u>Anthocyanins</u> are another family of amazing phytonutrients that provide the vibrant purple and blue color in many fruits and vegetables, including blueberries, cherries, purple grapes, purple eggplant, and pomegranates. Anthocyanins keep your brain sharp, help your heart and blood vessels stay healthy, and are powerful protectors of your cells from damage.

Sulforaphane is an amazing phytonutrient found in the cruciferous vegetable family, which consists of vegetables like broccoli, kale, Brussel sprouts, cabbage, and Bok choy. Sulforaphane is super powerful, and it's protective for heart health, brain health, liver health, and the health of all our cells.

So, phytonutrients are pretty amazing, and in order to optimize your health and feel your best, try to eat as many of these as possible! But how can we tell if we are eating foods that have lots of vitamins and minerals and phytonutrients?

The easiest way to identify food that that has a lot of micronutrients and phytonutrients is to eat fruits and vegetables which have lots of colors! The more colors you eat, and the more vibrant the colors, the more micronutrients and phytonutrients you will get.

A great strategy to get as many vitamins, minerals, and phytonutrients as possible is to try to "eat a rainbow" every day, or even better, at every meal. For example, to eat a rainbow you can eat red strawberries, orange sweet potatoes, yellow bananas, green spinach, blue blueberries, purple grapes, and white cauliflower.

Here is how eating these colors of the rainbow helps your body:

- Red foods (like strawberries, tomatoes, and red peppers): Help keep your heart healthy and protect your body from getting sick.
- Orange foods (like carrots, sweet potatoes, and oranges): Help your eyes stay sharp and your skin stay healthy.
- Yellow foods (like bananas, corn, and yellow peppers): Give you energy and help keep your nerves and muscles working well.
- Green foods (like spinach, broccoli, and green apples): Make your bones strong, help your body fight off sickness, and give you lots of energy.
- Blue and Purple foods (like blueberries, grapes, and eggplant): Help your brain stay smart, your memory strong, and protect your cells from damage.
- White foods (like cauliflower, mushrooms, and garlic): Help support your immune system and help you heal when you're sick.

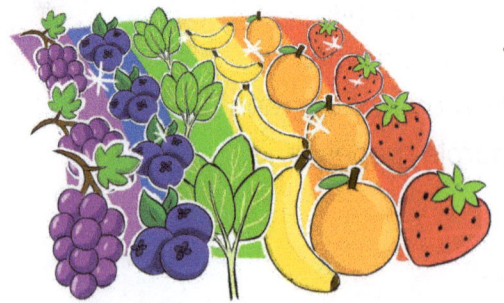

The food that nature made for us, the nutrients in that food, and our bodies are truly extraordinary!

PHYTONUTRIENT CHART

RED
Lycopene:
Protects your heart and helps keep your skin healthy.

  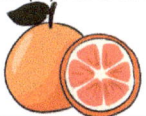

ORANGE
Beta-Carotene:
Keeps your eyes sharp and your immune system strong.

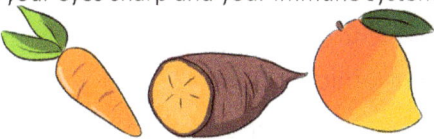

YELLOW
Lutein & Zeaxanthin:
Protect your eyes and help your brain stay sharp.

 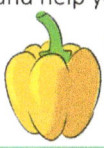 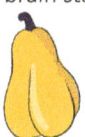

GREEN
Sulforaphane:
Protects your cells and helps your body get rid of harmful toxins.

 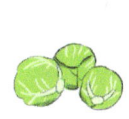 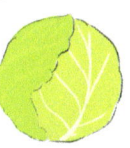

BLUE & PURPLE
Anthocyanins:
Help your memory and protect your brain.

WHITE
Allicin:
Boosts your immune system and helps fight germs.

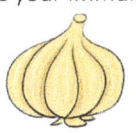 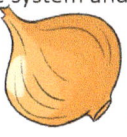 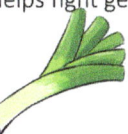

The Power of Micronutrients!

Did you know that according to scientific estimates, your body performs more than a billion billion chemical reactions every second? (No, that is not a typo! A billion billion, is another way of saying 1 billion times 1 billion, also known as 1 quintillion). And did you know that every single one of those chemical reactions requires vitamins and minerals?

Eat The Rainbow!

Unfortunately, most kids and adults don't eat enough micronutrients for their bodies to function at their best! This is because the packaged food from factories, which often makes up most of what people eat, does not contain a lot of these powerful micronutrients and phytonutrients. But when you eat lots of fruits and vegetables every day— foods made in nature that are loaded with vitamins, minerals, and phytonutrients—it helps your body function at its best. This can make a huge difference in how you grow and how you look and feel. This may include increasing your energy level, boosting your mood, and even improving the health of your skin, sometimes even in just a few days or weeks!

Challenge: Can you try eating a rainbow of colors at lunch every day this week?

CHAPTER 5
OUR FOOD IS FOOD FOR OUR GUT MICROBIOME

Did you know that when you eat, you are not just feeding yourself, but you are also feeding trillions of organisms that live inside your intestines? This may seem hard to believe, but on and inside your body there lives a gigantic community of bacteria, viruses, and fungi that have a big impact on your health. This community is called the <u>microbiome</u>.

Your microbiome is like a crowded city that lives on and inside of you! It is incredible!

Not just that, but also the size of your microbiome is mind blowing. It contains trillions of microorganisms. We have about the same number of microorganisms in and on our body than the number of our human cells. Amazingly— if you add up all of the microorganisms in and on your body, it would probably total about 2-5 pounds, which is about the weight of your brain!

So, our microbiome is a huge part of us, and every day scientists are learning more about its gigantic role in our health.

Most of the <u>microbes</u> in your body live in your digestive tract, specifically the large intestine, also known as your gut. These organisms are called your gut microbiome.

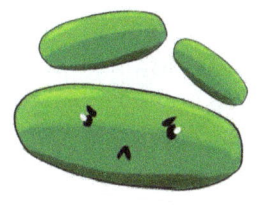

For most people, when we think about bacteria in our gut, we think about the bad bacteria that are sometimes found in rotten or contaminated food, like <u>Salmonella</u>, or E. coli. These bad bacteria can give you food poisoning and make you sick. But most of the bacteria that are living in your digestive tract are not harmful, and they don't make you sick. You actually need them to stay healthy.

So why is your gut microbiome so important? Let's talk about some of the ways that your gut microbiome impacts your health!

One important job is that the bacteria in your gut microbiome are crucial for your food digestion. The microbes break down complex carbohydrates, proteins, and some of the fats that reach the lower digestive tract. Your gut microbiome also helps your body produce some essential vitamins, which are necessary for good health. Not only that, but your gut microbiome also produces chemicals which help to feed the cells of your intestinal lining, to keep those cells in your digestive tract healthy and strong.

Our Microbiome and Micronutrients

Our gut microbiome helps us produce many important vitamins that are essential for our health! Some examples of these vitamins are: Vitamin B1 (Thiamine), Vitamin B2 (Riboflavin), Vitamin B12 (Cobalamin), and Vitamin K (Phylloquinone).

So, your gut microbiome is super important for your digestive system health and food digestion. But believe it or not, this is just the beginning! The microbiome in your gut does so much more than just aid with healthy digestion. Your microbiome actually has a big impact on many other parts of your body too.

Good bacteria in the microbiome are believed to strengthen our immune system, help us stay healthy and free from diseases, and even improve our brain function.

First let's talk about the connection with our immune system.

Every day, scientists are learning more about the connection between our microbiome and our immune system, and we know that our microbiome and our immune system are closely connected in several ways. First, the bacteria in our gut are the first line of defense in our intestinal tract. They are an important part of maintaining the intestinal barrier and protecting against the invasion of harmful bacteria.

Your microbiome is also important for training your immune system and helping it mature. When you are young, and your immune system is just developing, the presence of these organisms in your body helps to stimulate your immune system to make it stronger. But your microbiome may also make your immune system smarter too. When your immune system is exposed to the harmless organisms in your microbiome, it helps your immune system learn what organisms are harmless, and which ones are a threat.

These connections between your immune system and your microbiome may explain why your microbiome health has been linked with the health of your digestive tract, and even with conditions like allergies and asthma, which are linked with your immune system.

Next, let's look at the effect of your microbiome on your brain.

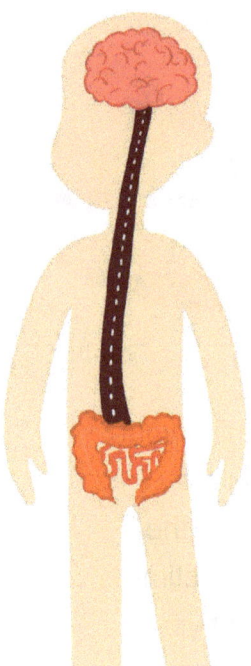

The gut-brain connection is the term to describe the partnership between your digestive tract and your brain. Imagine that in your body, there are highways that connect different parts of it, so that your organs can communicate. One of the most important highways is between your digestive tract (gut) and your brain. This highway is used all day long to send messages back and forth between your digestive tract and brain. Some people even refer to our digestive tract as a second brain, because it produces many of the same chemicals that send messages in the brain (called neurotransmitters). These neurotransmitters, including serotonin, dopamine, and GABA are all involved in regulating your mood and your mental health.

Have You Ever Felt "Hangry"?

The term "hangry" is sometimes used to describe the feeling of becoming angry when you feel really hungry. This feeling of being hangry is likely not a coincidence and is one example of the gut brain connection. When your digestive tract senses a lack of food, it sends a signal to your brain that triggers hunger. For some people though, these signals may also trigger a feeling of irritability or mood changes.

Our microbiome is a big part of the gut brain connection, and scientists believe that changes in our gut microbiome can alter our brain chemistry. There have even been several studies that suggest that the gut microbiome may be related to our mood, our ability to concentrate, and our memory. For example, when your gut microbiome is healthy and happy, it can send signals to your brain, so you feel happy and relaxed. On the other hand, when your gut microbiome is unhealthy, it can send signals to your brain that can make you feel sad or anxious.

So, with all of this being said, with a healthy gut microbiome being linked with fewer stomachaches, a stronger and smarter immune system, better concentration, and feeling happier, let's talk about how you can boost your microbiome health!

The most important way to improve your microbiome health is to feed the microbes in your gut their favorite food! The number one favorite food for your microbiome is fiber.

Fiber is a type of complex carbohydrate that is only found in plants, such as fruits and vegetables. Unlike most of the nutrients that humans eat, fiber cannot be broken down and absorbed by our digestive tract, which makes it available for our microbiome as their preferred food source. Fiber also helps to support our digestive tract, helping us poop, so we get fewer stomachaches.

Good sources of fiber include fruits, vegetables, whole grains (such as 100% whole grain bread, brown rice, and oatmeal), beans, lentils, nuts, and seeds.

Sadly though, most children and adults in the U.S. don't eat nearly enough fiber, because they don't eat enough plants. Most fast food, and most of the food that is made in factories and found in packages do not contain a lot of fiber or nutrients. To eat enough fiber to support the health of your microbiome and digestive tract, it is best to eat plants (fruits and vegetables, beans, lentils, nuts, seeds, and whole grains) every day and at every meal!

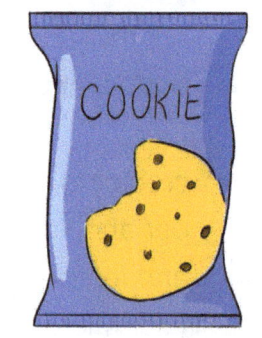

When you eat fiber at every meal, it helps the microbes in your gut become healthy and flourish! Healthy microbes can then produce chemicals that benefit your health! This relationship is a win-win. When your microbes are happy and healthy, they help you feel happy and healthy too!

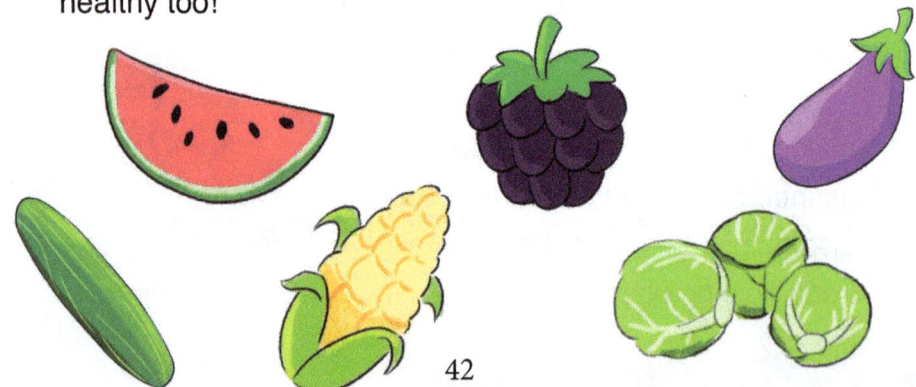

Are there any foods that our microbiome doesn't like?

Yes! Gut microbes do not like a lot of the artificial sweeteners, artificial colors, and artificial flavors that are found in some packaged foods made in factories.

Eating too much sugar is also unhealthy for our gut microbes. When we eat too much sugar, it harms the healthy gut bacteria and instead feeds the unhealthy gut microbes. When this happens, our microbiome can be thrown out of balance, with less healthy gut bacteria and more harmful microbes. This has a negative impact on our health.

So bottom line, our food is incredible, and so is our microbiome! When you eat foods with lots of fiber, which is naturally found in foods like fruits, vegetables, beans, lentils, nuts, seeds, whole grains, and other plants, you will help your microbiome thrive, which in turn will help you thrive!

CHAPTER 6
OUR FOOD IS INSTRUCTIONS AND INFORMATION

Did you know that your body has a personalized instruction manual? This instruction manual is a guide that tells your body exactly how it's supposed to work, and provides detailed, step by step instructions on how to build and run your body. These instructions come from your parents and stay the same throughout your life.

What? You don't believe it? You don't think this could be true? You have never seen your instruction manual?

Well, it is true, and the reason you haven't seen it is because your personalized instruction manual is too small to be seen by your eyes! The instruction manual is found in each and every one of the cells in your body, and it is called your DNA.

DNA, which stands for Deoxyribonucleic Acid, is

like a set of instructions that tells your body how to grow, develop, and function. Your DNA instructions are the foundation of who you are, from the color of your hair and skin to how your body operates.

Inside the instruction manual (your DNA), there are thousands of specific sections of instructions called genes. Each gene is a single section of the manual that provides a code of instructions that tells your body how to make a specific part of you or how to do a particular job in your body. For example, one gene could be the instructions for how to build the color of your eyes, while another gene could provide the instructions that determine your hair color, or the length of your toes. Genes are amazing!

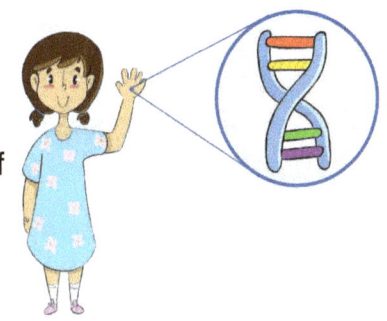

For a long time, doctors and scientists believed that your genes determined your future, and that you had no control over what your genes told your body to do. But now we know that's not entirely true.

Did you know that the food you eat can influence how your genes work?

If you imagine your DNA as the instruction manual and your genes as specific instructions, the food you eat can act as a highlighter to mark which areas of the instruction manual should be used by your body. These highlighter marks don't change what the instruction manual says, but they can help your body focus on certain parts of the instructions more than others. The highlighter marks from the food you eat can even turn certain instructions (genes) on and off.

This phenomenon-- that the food you eat and the way you live affects which genes are turned on and off, and how your genes work-- is called epigenetics.

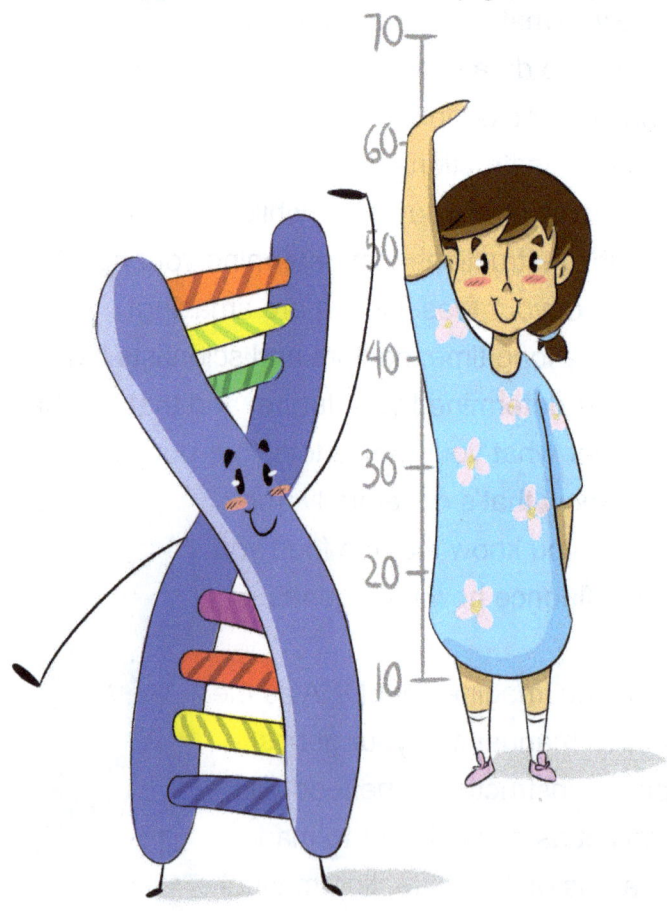

Here is an example. Imagine that you are growing taller every year, thanks to a set of genes that determines how tall you will be. While your genes provide the instructions for how tall you might grow, the food you eat helps your body follow those instructions in the best way possible, through epigenetics.

By eating foods which are rich in micronutrients (with lots of colors of the rainbow) and eating adequate protein (including lean meats, beans, lentils, nuts, and seeds), you are sending signals to your body to turn on the genes that support muscle and bone growth and development. In this way, the food you eat can send messages to your body that help make the most of your genetic potential for height, allowing you to grow as tall and strong as possible!

Not only that, but more and more, doctors and scientists are learning that through epigenetic changes, the food we eat has the potential to turn genes on and off, genes that can determine how long we live and our risk for many of the world's most common diseases.

For example, by making healthy food choices now, you can influence the instruction manual that determines your health for the rest of your life, decrease your risk for diseases as you get older, and potentially add years to your life!

On the other hand, eating too much sugar or eating foods that are lacking nutrients, (like many packaged foods made in factories, including candy, chips, or soda) can cause unhealthy marks on your DNA. These marks may turn on genes that lead to developing more diseases as you get older. It's like putting a mark on your instruction manual that says, "Turn on this unhealthy gene" or "Don't pay attention to this important step."

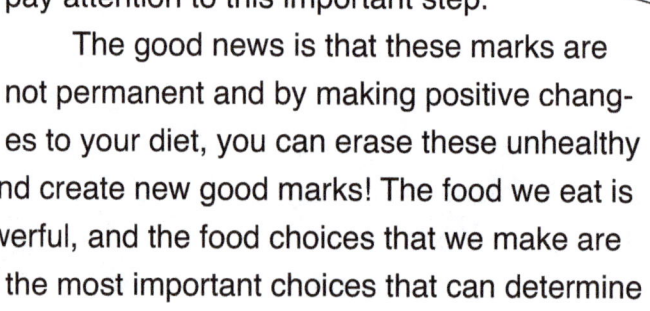

The good news is that these marks are not permanent and by making positive changes to your diet, you can erase these unhealthy marks and create new good marks! The food we eat is truly powerful, and the food choices that we make are some of the most important choices that can determine our future!

The way that food influences our epigenetics is just one important way that food acts as information or instructions. But believe it or not, there are even more examples of how the food we eat acts as information, that are just as surprising and amazing!

With every bite of food that we eat, our stomach and digestive tract send signals all over our body, telling our body what to do and feel and what hormones (chemical messengers) to produce. These messages in turn set off processes for different things to happen in your body.

In Chapter 2, we talked about how calories are just a measure of energy, and that calories don't tell us the quality of the energy in food. We talked about how when we eat simple carbohydrates, our body can break them down very quickly and we get a quick spike of energy and then a crash. On the other hand, when we eat complex carbohydrates like fruits, vegetables, beans, lentils, and whole grains, we get sustained good energy that lasts.

There is another reason why focusing on the calorie content of food is misleading, and it has to do with the information and messages that our food sends to our body!

This is especially important to understand for many adults who are struggling to lose weight by counting calories. Sadly, most adults have never been taught why our food is so incredible, why our food choices are so important, and why just looking at calories is so misleading.

Unfortunately, the weight loss business makes this problem worse. The weight loss business is made up of companies that sell products, programs, and advice to help people lose weight. Many of these companies sell diets, pills, powders, and shakes that promise quick weight loss, and they make billions of dollars per year! But rather than teaching people how to feel stronger and healthier with the amazing power of food, a lot of these companies offer bad advice that tricks people. Not only that, but most of the time the weight loss business focuses only on numbers— like how much someone weighs or how many calories they eat.

But, as we have learned, our bodies and our food are incredible! True health isn't just about how much we weigh! And the food we eat is so much more than just calories!

Whenever you eat, your stomach and digestive track send information and messages all over your body, which then set off processes for different things to happen in your body. These processes determine how hungry you feel, and whether you gain or lose weight.

Let's look at an example.

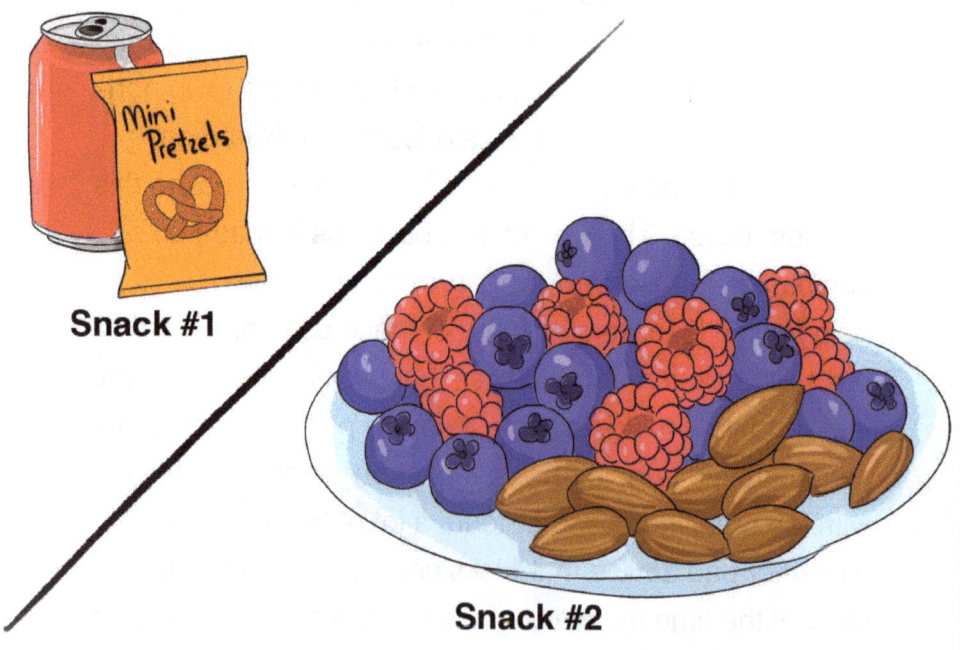

Snack #1

Snack #2

Imagine that an adult is trying to lose weight, and they want to have a snack. There are two options. The first is a diet soda and a snack sized package of mini pretzels. The diet soda is 0 calories, and the package of mini pretzels is 100 calories. The other option is a big plate full of blueberries and raspberries, and two handfuls of almonds. This second snack option is about 350 calories.

For many adults who are on a diet and counting calories, they may choose snack #1 because it has fewer calories. They have also been told by food companies that these "low calorie" or "no calorie" foods are good for weight loss.

But guess which snack is better for someone who wants to lose weight?

Snack #2 is the better choice— even though it has more than 3 times the number of calories! The reason that snack #2 is a better choice is because of the positive information and messages those foods send to your body.

Let's look at this a little closer to understand why.

When you have the diet soda and package of pretzels, your stomach and intestines break down the pretzels almost immediately. The pretzels are an example of simple or refined carbohydrates without any fiber or nutrients. Similar to many other packaged foods made in factories, we know that once the pretzels are quickly digested, it causes a quick rise of your blood sugar. This quick steep rise in your blood sugar is a message that triggers your pancreas to secrete a burst of insulin. Insulin is a hormone (a chemical messenger) that causes you to store the extra sugar as fat, so you can use that sugar later.

Now let's talk about the diet soda. The diet soda contains artificial sweeteners to make it taste sweet, and we know that artificial chemicals including artificial sweeteners are harmful for our microbiome. Scientists have also found that artificial sweeteners can send messages to people's brains to make them crave more food and sugar.

Not only that, but within a few minutes of eating the diet soda and pretzels snack, your stomach is empty, and through your gut-brain connection, your stomach sends a message to your brain that it is empty and that you need more food! So even though you just had a snack, you are hungry again!

So bottom line, with snack #1, even though the food is only 100 calories, it has sent messages to make your body to store sugar as fat, crave more sugar, and feel hungry! Not only that, but this snack has little to no micronutrients, will not give you good lasting energy, and is not healthy for your microbiome.

Now that look at what happens with the snack of nuts and berries. Remember this snack has over three times the calories!

Almonds and berries are both foods made in nature, that are naturally filled with fiber and lots of micronutrients and phytonutrients.

When you eat the almonds, the natural fiber slows down their digestion, so the energy is released more gradually. You won't have the quick blood sugar spike and crash, and instead you will have lasting, sustained good energy. Because you won't have the big sharp spike in your blood sugar, your pancreas will not get the message to release a burst of insulin.

The berries are similar. Because the berries are rich in fiber, micronutrients, and phytonutrients, they will give you stable, sustained energy, without causing a big spike in your blood sugar and without triggering your body to have a big spike in its insulin level.

Not only that, but because the almonds and berries are full of fiber, it will take time for your stomach to digest this snack, and your stomach will feel full longer. Through your gut brain connection, your brain will get a message that you feel satisfied and full.

Even better, with the snack of almonds and berries, you are helping to keep your microbiome healthy, and all the micronutrients and phytonutrients are helping your cells stay healthy!

So bottom line, with snack #2, even though the nuts and berries are over 3 times the calories, it has sent messages to your body so you feel full and satisfied, you have stable and sustained good energy, your microbiome is happy, and your cells are happy.

This is just one example of why calorie counting is not a good idea. More important than the number of calories, it is the quality of what we are eating that matters.

So next time you are having a snack, what will you choose? If you choose foods from nature that are filled with nutrients, rather than packaged food from factories, you will be sending positive messages to your entire body! There are so many delicious foods to choose from.

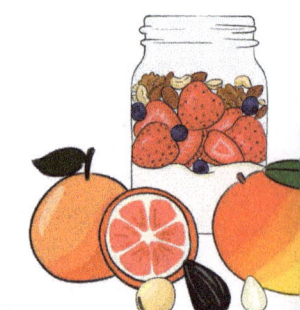

Here are some great snack ideas:
- Whole fruit
- Nuts, nut butters
- Plain yogurt, with or without your own fruit added
- Seeds, seed butters
- Carrots or cucumbers with hummus

Food is so much more than just calories!

Remember, rather than focusing on numbers on a scale and numbers of calories, it is more important to focus on nourishing ourselves with the extraordinary food that nature has created for us.

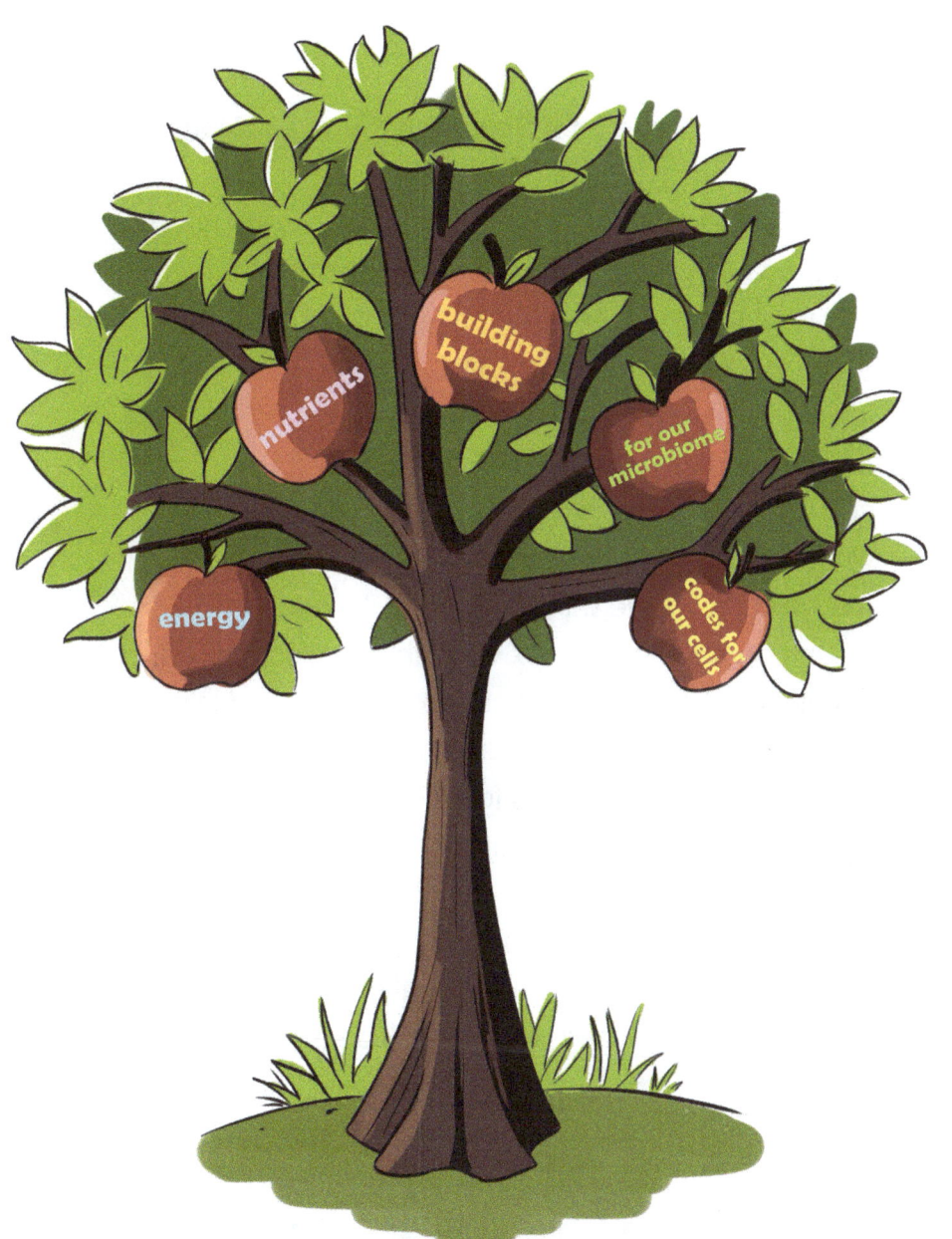

Food is energy.
Food is nutrients that allow our cells to function.
Food is the building blocks of our body.
Food is food for our microbiome.
Food is messages/codes for our cells.

Are Numbers on a Scale the Same as Health?

With all that we have learned so far, we know that our food is so much more than just calories! For many adults who have never learned about food, they think that just looking at the number of calories in food is the best way to see if it's a healthy choice. But if we just look at the number of calories in food, we will miss all 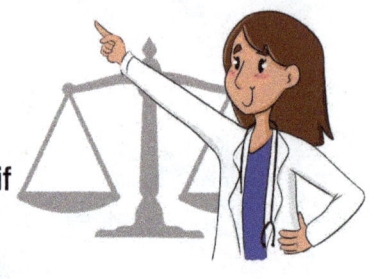 the important and complex ways that the food we eat is connected to the health of our bodies. Our food is our energy. Our food is our building blocks. Our food is our micronutrients. Our food is food for our microbiome. And our food is messages for our cells. Our food is truly incredible!

But how about our bodies? They are incredible and complex too! Sadly, many adults have never learned much about this either. Sometimes adults think that being healthy is just about what the scale says. That's the number you see when someone steps on it and it shows how much they weigh.

But just like calories don't tell us the whole story about food, numbers on a scale don't tell us the whole story about our health.

Your body is so much more than a number!
Let's look at a pretend example:

Imagine two people who weigh the exact same amount. One of them didn't eat much for a few weeks because they were trying to lose weight. When they did eat, they mostly ate fast food and snacks from packages. They felt really tired and didn't move their body much.

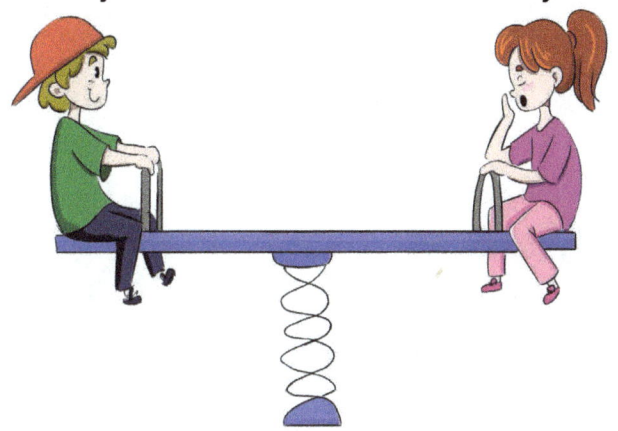

The other person learned about the power of food and started eating more fruits, veggies, healthy proteins, healthy fats, and whole grains. They lost weight too, but they felt full of energy, and they felt strong! They had fun playing outside and moving their body. They even felt more confident and happier.

Even though they both weigh the same, the one who ate healthier foods and felt stronger and happier is likely much healthier on the inside! What really matters is how you feel, how your body works, and how you take care of yourself—not just a number on a scale.

If you are trying to improve your health, rather than focusing on numbers on a scale, a better approach is to focus on nourishing yourself with healthy food.

PART 3:
OUR EARTH IS
EXTRAORDINARY

CHAPTER 7
CHOOSING EXTRAORDINARY FOOD

Have you ever heard the phrase, "Knowledge is power?" This means when you gain information and learn new things, it gives you the ability to make good choices and have more control over what happens in your life. When it comes to learning about food and your health, this could not be more true!

Now that we understand all the ways that food impacts the way that our body works, we can choose to eat foods that will help our bodies function at their best. This way, we will have more control over how we feel and more control over our future! Let's summarize some of the key concepts from what we learned, so we can figure out how to make good food choices.

- ✅ We want to eat mostly complex carbohydrates, so we can get lasting sustained energy.
- ✅ We want to eat healthy fats and protein, including monounsaturated fats and <u>omega 3 fats</u> to strengthen our bodies and our brains.
- ✅ We want to eat lots of micronutrients and phytonutrients, so that all of our cells can function at their best.
- ✅ We want to eat lots of fiber, so our microbiome is healthy and happy, so we feel healthier and happier too.
- ✅ We want to eat food that sends good messages to our cells and genes, which will benefit our health now and also in the future.

This may seem complicated. But, fortunately, it's not as complicated as it may sound. Thankfully, our Earth has made it easy for us!

Not only is food extraordinary, but our Earth is extraordinary too! When we eat the foods that the Earth has created for us, it will automatically help us follow all of these principles.

The foods that the Earth created for us are called whole foods. Whole foods are foods that come from plants and animals, that are eaten as close as possible to their natural state. Examples of whole foods are fruits, vegetables, beans, lentils, lean meats, milk, eggs, whole grains, nuts, and seeds. All of these foods are made by nature, rather than in factories, and these are the foods that the Earth intended for us to eat. Whole foods are extraordinary!

When you eat mostly whole foods, this will help your body function at its best. Let's look a little deeper and see how eating mostly whole foods can help you.

- ☑ When you eat whole food sources of carbohydrates, including fruits, vegetables, beans, lentils, and whole grains, you are eating mostly complex carbohydrates that will give you lasting sustained energy.
- ☑ When you eat whole food sources of protein and fat, including fish, lean meats, eggs, beans, lentils, nuts, avocados, olives, and seeds, you will be getting the healthy proteins you need to build muscle, but you will also be getting the healthy fats that are important for your brain.
- ☑ When you eat whole foods including lots of fruits and vegetables, you will be eating food with loads of micronutrients and phytonutrients. These micronutrients will help your body function at its best.
- ☑ When you eat whole foods, including fruits, vegetables, beans, lentils, whole grains, nuts, and seeds, you will be eating lots of fiber, which will help nourish your microbiome, which will help you stay healthy.

☑ When you eat whole foods, you will be sending good messages to your genes and your cells.

Whole foods, the foods that the Earth has created for us, are truly incredible!

The opposite of a whole food is an ultra-processed food. Ultra-processed foods are foods that are made in factories, which bear little resemblance to food found in nature. These are foods that are most often stripped of their fiber, stripped of their nutrients, and often contain lots of ingredients that are not found in nature. For many ultra-processed foods, when you look at the label, the ingredients may sound like they were made in a chemistry lab, and they often contain ingredients that you would not find in a normal kitchen.

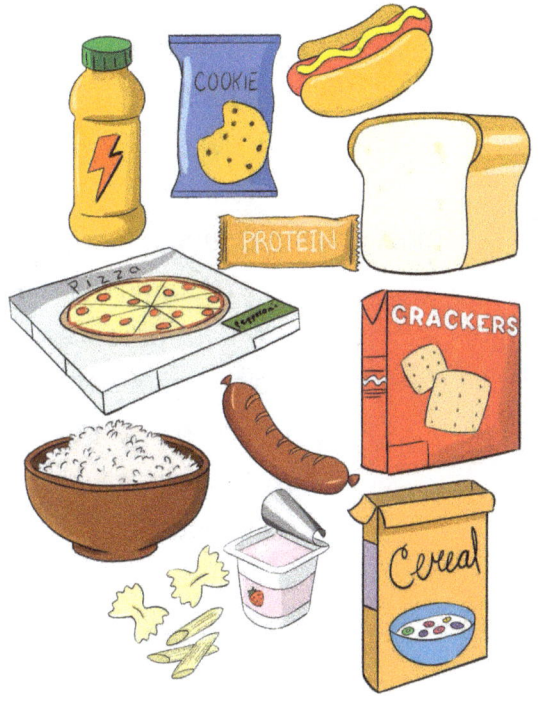

Sadly, most fast food and most food in our grocery stores is ultra-processed food. For this reason, most of the food that adults and kids in the U.S. are eating is ultra-processed food. It has been estimated that ultra-processed foods make up about 60% of what American adults eat and about 70% of what American kids eat. This is not good for us or good for our health.

Examples of ultra-processed foods are most packaged snack foods (including packaged cookies, bars, and crackers), most breakfast cereals, most frozen meals (like frozen pizza), refined grains (including white bread, white rice, and white pasta), processed meats (like hot dogs and sausage), flavored yogurts, sports drinks, and more.

Even though ultra-processed foods are some of the most commonly eaten foods in the world, ultra-processed foods are not extraordinary, like the foods found in nature.

- ☒ Many ultra-processed foods are made with simple sugars and refined carbohydrates, which provide energy, but not the stable, sustained energy that come with complex carbohydrates and whole foods.
- ☒ Many ultra-processed foods contain more of the unhealthier fats and less of the healthy fats and protein.
- ☒ Most ultra-processed foods are stripped of their nutrients, so they don't give your body the nutrients it needs to function at its best.
- ☒ Most ultra-processed foods are lacking fiber.
- ☒ Most ultra-processed foods contain ingredients like too much sugar, too much sodium (salt), or artificial flavors and colors that are unhealthy for our microbiome.
- ☒ Eating too much ultra-processed food can also

send unhealthy messages to your genes and cells, which can impact your health in the future.

If whole foods are so much healthier for us, why are people eating so much ultra-processed food?

Sadly, most of the food in our grocery stores and in our restaurants are ultra-processed foods. This is because food companies can make a lot more money selling ultra-processed foods than they can selling whole foods.

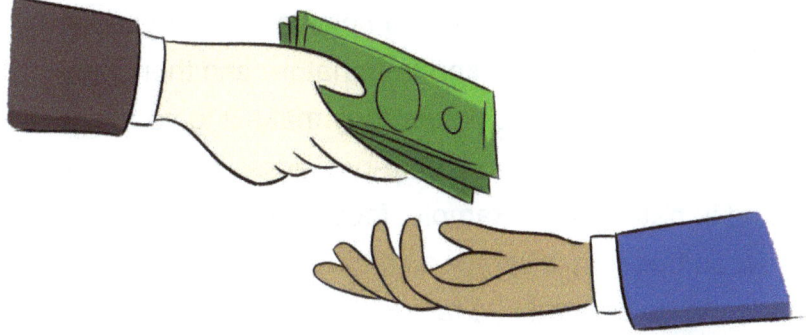

Ultra-processed foods are typically much less expensive to make because they are often made using artificially created ingredients that are less expensive for food manufacturers. Not only that, but many of these ultra-processed foods were intentionally designed by food manufacturers to contain ingredients (too much sugar, too much sodium, and unhealthy fats), which send messages to our bodies and brains that make us hungrier and crave more ultra-processed foods. This helps the food industry make even more money, because when we are hungrier and crave these ultra-processed foods, we buy more, and their profits increase.

So how can we recognize the difference between

whole foods and ultra-processed foods?

Whole foods are foods that are found in nature, that are processed as little as possible and are similar to what they are like in their natural state. This includes fruits, vegetables, beans, lentils, lean meats, eggs, dairy, nuts, and seeds. For example, when we eat an apple, we know exactly where that comes from in nature— an apple tree. Similarly, beans, nuts, and seeds grow on plants. All of these foods, whole foods, are taken from nature and then there is very little that changes before they make it to your plate.

On the other hand, ultra-processed foods are not found in nature. For example, foods like crackers don't grow on trees. In order for a cracker to get to your plate, it needs to be created in a factory by combining a variety of ingredients and making a dough. Then the dough must be rolled out and shaped and cut. Lastly, the shaped dough must be cooked and packaged. This process is called food processing, where raw ingredients (whole foods) are changed into different food products using mechanical and chemical methods.

But not all crackers are ultra-processed foods— some crackers are processed more or less than others. For example, some crackers are made with just a few ingredients, and all of the ingredients are whole foods. To make these crackers, there is some processing that is required (mixing the few ingredients, rolling, baking, cutting), but it is not a lot of processing.

Some crackers are ultra-processed, meaning there is a lot of processing required to make them. These crackers may have a long list of ingredients, and the ingredients may not be whole foods from nature (or even typically found in a normal kitchen). Instead, the list of ingredients may contain lots of added ingredients that you may not 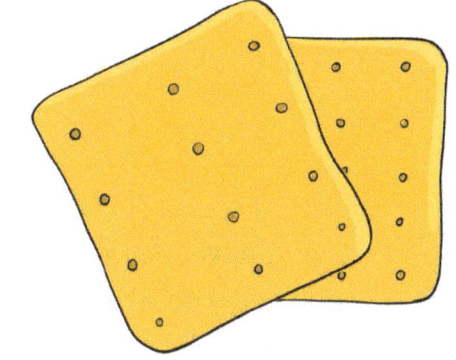 recognize, including preservatives, artificial colors, artificial flavors, added sweeteners, or added oils. For example, in crackers that are ultra-processed, some of the ingredients may even sound like they were created in a chemistry lab, not a kitchen!

The most important way to tell if a food is processed a little bit (slightly processed or moderately processed), versus ultra-processed is to look at the ingredients. If there is a long list of ingredients, or if the ingredient list contains chemicals or words you don't recognize, it is most likely an ultra-processed food. Not only that, but ultra-processed foods are also mostly found in plastic packages. On the other hand, whole foods (for example, foods like apples and broccoli) often don't need to be in a plastic package.

> **Pop Quiz!**
>
> Question: What is the most important thing to look for when reading food labels?...
>
> Answer: No label at all! (That means it probably grew from the Earth, not a factory!) 🤣
>
> The food that we want to be eating the most is food that doesn't have labels. When you eat foods like fresh fruits and vegetables, they don't have labels, because you know exactly what they are. **They are a food found in nature that nature intended us to eat.**

Ideally, when we are choosing foods to eat, it is best to choose mostly whole foods. Then if we choose to eat foods like crackers that are processed, it is best to choose crackers that have been only slightly processed, rather than choosing the ultra-processed kinds.

How can we make better choices and eat more whole foods and less ultra-processed food?

Ultra-processed food is everywhere, and some ultra-processed foods may be some of the foods that we are used to eating and may even enjoy the most! This is especially true because food manufacturers have intentionally created ultra-processed food to send messages to our taste buds and our brains, so they may seem irresistible!

Have you ever finished eating a snack sized package of chips and then wanted a second bag? This is because the chips were intentionally designed to send messages to your body, to make you crave more!

For this reason, it is not easy to completely avoid ultra-processed food. But even if we can increase the amount of whole foods that we are eating while we reduce the amount of ultra-processed food that we are eating, this is a great first step!

Rather than focusing on **CUTTING OUT** the ultra-processed foods, a better approach is to focus on **CROWDING OUT** the ultra-processed foods. **CROWDING OUT** means, if you focus on trying to eat more or mostly whole foods, you will naturally have less room on your plate and in your stomach for the processed foods. Similarly, when you choose to eat something processed, if you try to choose more slightly processed foods, you will have less room on your plate for the ultra-processed foods.

Your brain will help you with this too. The more whole foods and slightly processed foods you eat, the less you will crave the other stuff.

For example, maybe you can start by reaching for an apple and peanut butter for a snack, instead of reaching for a bag of chips or crackers. After you eat the apple and peanut butter, you may not be as hungry for the chips and crackers.

Or perhaps for breakfast, you can choose a bowl of rolled oats (oatmeal) with berries and nuts, rather than eating a bowl of sweet cereal. After you eat the oats, berries, and nuts, which are loaded with fiber and nutrients, you may not be hungry for the bowl of sweet cereal.

Or maybe if you feel like eating cheese and crackers, you can look at the ingredients on the box of crackers, and choose crackers made with just whole grains, seeds, and spices, rather than the crackers with a long list of ingredients.

When you eat more whole foods, this will automatically help you eat less ultra-processed food! The idea is not to feel bad if you eat ultra-processed food sometimes, but to feel good that you are eating more whole foods!

Then if you start eating more whole foods and less ultra-processed foods by crowding out, you may even start noticing an improvement in how you feel. This could include increased energy, an improved mood, improved digestion, less stomachaches, or even a clearer complexion. When you start noticing that you feel better, this can help you crave the whole foods and crowd out the ultra-processed foods even more!

Our Earth, and the whole foods that our Earth created for us, are extraordinary!

Don't be Fooled by the Health Halo

Have you ever seen a food that looks healthy… but then find out that it actually isn't the best choice? That's something called the health halo effect!

A halo is a glowing circle you sometimes see drawn around people's heads in cartoons or pictures to show that they're good. The health halo is when a food seems healthy—because of the way it's packaged, labeled, or advertised—even if it's not the best choice.

For example, if a snack says "low fat," "natural," or "gluten-free," some people might think it's super healthy—without actually looking at what's really inside. But guess what? That same snack might still be full of sugar, artificial ingredients, or barely any nutrients at all. That's the health halo tricking us!

The best way to know if something is actually healthy is to look closely at the ingredients and ask, "Is this a whole food? "Is it full of good stuff like fiber or nutrients?" "Does this have lots of ultra-processed ingredients like sugar, salt, or added oils?"

For example: Imagine you see a granola bar that says "All Natural" and "Made with whole grains!" This may sound good, right? But then if you check the ingredients, you may see it's made with lots of sugar, mostly refined grains, barely any fiber, and lots of words you can't pronounce. That's the health halo at work!

Don't let the health halo fool you—just because something looks or sounds healthy, doesn't mean it always is!

Corn and Ultra-Processed Food

Did you know that ingredients made from corn are some of the most common ingredients in ultra-processed food? This may sound healthy— but unfortunately, it's not! Eating whole, unprocessed corn like corn on the cob is wonderful! Whole corn is a complex carbohydrate, and eating it will provide stable, good energy. It also contains fiber, vitamins, minerals, and even healthy phytonutrients.

On the other hand, the corn ingredients that are used in most ultra-processed foods are different. To create the corn ingredients used in ultra-processed food, the corn gets taken to a factory, and the food manufacturers use chemicals and machines to take the corn kernels apart and remake the corn into other ingredients. These ingredients no longer look like corn, and they no longer have the fiber and nutrients in the original corn. These ultra-processed corn-derived ingredients are also no longer healthy like corn.

Once you recognize the ultra-processed ingredients made from corn, and you start looking closely at the ingredients on food labels, you will see that these corn-based ingredients are in almost everything processed!

Corn and Ultra-Processed Food

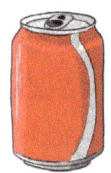

- Most sodas are made mostly of corn in the form of <u>high fructose corn syrup</u>.
- Many ultra-processed breakfast cereals are made mostly of corn: corn flour and <u>corn starch</u>, with more corn on top, in the form of high fructose corn syrup.
- Most candy is also made from corn, with some of the most common ingredients being high fructose corn syrup, corn starch, and maltodextrin (another form of sugar), which are all made of corn.
- Many chips and snacks are made with corn flour or fried with corn oil.

Unfortunately, ultra-processed corn ingredients are everywhere! Some ultra-processed ingredients made from corn:

- High fructose corn syrup
- <u>Dextrose</u>
- Corn starch
- Corn oil
- <u>Erythritol</u>
- <u>Xanthan gum</u>

So why is there corn in everything? Corn is inexpensive— mostly because the U.S. government pays farmers to grow lots of it. Because of this, food companies, who are interested in making more money, have learned how to use corn as a substitute for whole food ingredients.

The Truth About Sugar

Did you know that most ultra-processed foods have added sugar—even foods you wouldn't expect? Often foods that aren't supposed to be sweet, like crackers, pasta sauces, and bread have a lot of added sugar. The term 'added sugar' refers to sugar that is added in addition to the sugar that naturally occurs in the food. One example is applesauce. Apples naturally contain sugar, but some manufacturers add more sugar to make applesauce.

And the foods that are supposed to be sweet, like packaged cookies, sweetened yogurts, and granola bars—well most of those have been made to taste super sweet, with a lot more sugar in them than is needed. Not only that, but drinks like soda, sports drinks, and even juice are filled with sugar!

This is because food companies have learned that when they put a lot of sugar in their food products, it makes people crave their products more. Then when people buy more of their products, they can make more money!

This is why most adults and kids in the U.S. eat about 17 teaspoons of added sugar every day! That adds up to around 60 pounds of added sugar every year. (That is about three super full backpacks filled with books!) Most people have no idea they are eating (and drinking) that much sugar!

This is important because, as we have learned, too much sugar can mess with your energy level, hurt your microbiome, and send unhealthy messages to your cells.

The Truth About Sugar

Are artificial sweeteners any better? Artificial sweeteners are fake sugars that are created in a chemistry lab to replace regular sugar. Some food companies make it seem like these sweeteners are a healthy choice, but they can actually be harmful for our bodies. These fake sugars can trick your brain into wanting more sweets, send confusing signals to your body's cells, and even hurt your gut microbiome.

How can you spot added sugar and artificial sweeteners? The best way is to look at the ingredient list! Sugar and artificial sweeteners can hide under names like:

• Agave nectar	• Fruit juice concentrates
• Corn syrup	• High fructose corn syrup
• Dextrose	• Honey
• Evaporated cane juice	• Maltose
• Fructose	• Sucrose
• <u>Aspartame</u>, <u>sucralose</u>, <u>sorbitol</u>, <u>mannitol</u>, <u>xylitol</u>, and <u>saccharin</u> (these are artificial sweeteners!)	

While eating some sugar is ok sometimes, it is best to aim to eat mostly whole foods with natural sweetness, like fruit! At first, eating fruit may not taste as sweet as eating ultra-processed foods with added sugars or artificial sweeteners. But the more you crowd out the added sugar and artificial sweeteners, the more your taste buds will start to appreciate the natural sweetness of foods made in nature (like blueberries, raspberries, watermelon, carrots, apples, and mangos)! Your body and your gut bugs will thank you!

CHAPTER 8
CREATING AN INCREDIBLE PLATE

Now that we have talked about the extraordinary power of whole foods, let's put it all together, and see what healthy eating looks like on your plate!

Here is what you can aim for:

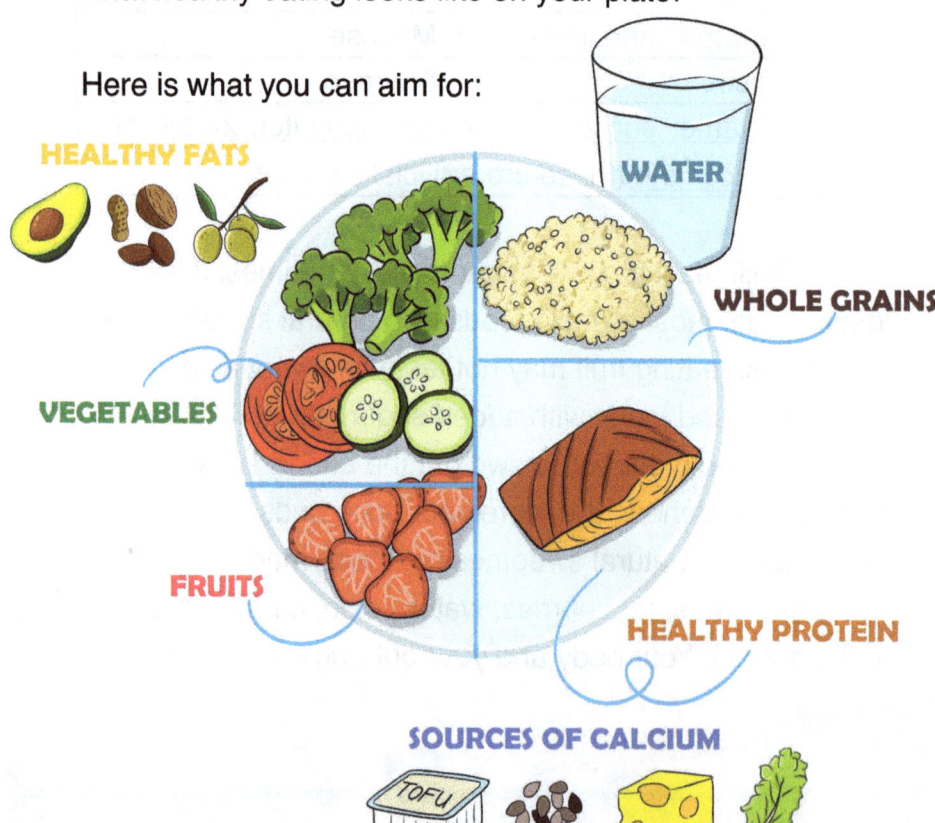

- ✅ For every meal, try to make half of your plate fruits and vegetables! Choose a variety of vegetables and whole fruits with lots of different colors! By doing this, you will be eating lots of fiber, micronutrients, phytonutrients, and healthy carbohydrates. (Please note that potatoes are in the grain category, and that drinking fruit juice does not count as eating fruit.)
- ✅ For every meal, make one quarter of your plate healthy proteins. The healthiest sources of protein are beans, lentils, nuts, seeds, fish, eggs, and lean meats like chicken breast. Aim to eat these healthier sources of protein in place of red meat and processed meats such as hot dogs and sausage, which are not as healthy for your body. Eating protein at every meal is important because when we eat enough protein, we are giving our bodies what we need to build new cells and build muscle.
- ✅ Make one quarter of your plate whole grains. This includes foods like rolled oats, brown rice, whole grain pasta, quinoa, and whole wheat bread, rather than white rice, white pasta, or white bread. Eating whole grains is

important, because whole grains are a healthy source of complex carbohydrates that will give us sustained energy. Whole grains will also provide nutrients and fiber for our microbiome.

☑ Include healthy fats to your diet every day. Examples are foods like nuts, seeds, olives, avocados, and certain types of fish like salmon. This is important because healthy fats are important for our cell and brain health.

☑ Drink water, as the drink of choice with every meal or snack, rather than drinking juice or sugary beverages. Water is the best choice for quenching your thirst.

☑ Try to include some foods on your plate that are a good source of calcium. This could include dairy products such as milk, yogurt, or cheese, which are whole foods and good sources of the mineral calcium. There are also other great options to get calcium that are not dairy products, including dark green leafy vegetables like kale, almonds, chia seeds, tofu, or organic soy milk.

Let's look at some examples of incredible plates.

For Breakfast:

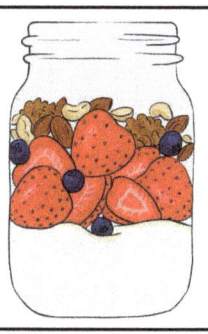	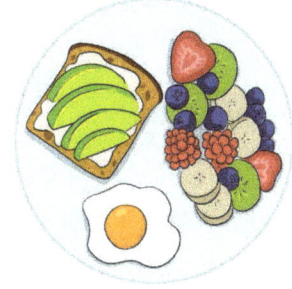
Plain yogurt with nuts, lots of berries.	A bowl of fruit with a piece of whole grain avocado toast and an egg.

For Lunch:

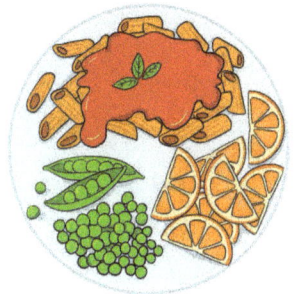	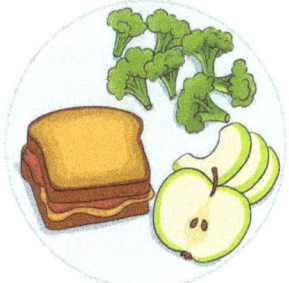
Lentil pasta and sauce, peas, oranges	Peanut butter and low-sugar jam sandwich on whole grain bread, broccoli and an apple

For Dinner:

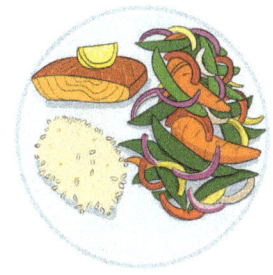	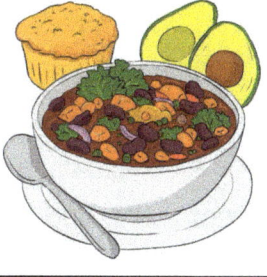
Grilled salmon with brown rice, vegetable stir fry with green beans, bell peppers, onions, and carrots	Vegetarian chili with black beans, kidney beans, carrots, onions, bell peppers, and kale. Served with whole grain cornbread & avocado.

Drinking Water For The Win!

Did you know that your body is made mostly of water? And did you know that drinking water, rather than juice, sports drinks, or sodas, is one of the best things you can do for your body?

Water is important to:
- Stay hydrated so you have energy
- Take care of your brain so you can think clearly and remember things
- Keep your body cool when you're running and playing sports
- Support your digestion (so you poop regularly!)
- Maintain blood flow, so your immune system and cells can work properly

What About Soda Or Sports Drinks?

These drinks might taste good, but they are typically made of sugar or artificial sweeteners, and artificial colors and flavors that come from factories and chemistry labs, not from our Earth. As we have learned, these ingredients can all harm our microbiome and send unhealthy messages to our cells.

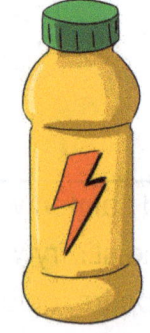

What About Juice?

Even though a glass of fruit juice may sound healthy, it contains lots of sugar too! Even if this sugar is natural sugar (not added sugar), it still counts as sugar. Drinking fruit juice is different than eating whole fruit (a whole food), because the sugar in whole fruit is naturally packaged with the fiber and nutrients in the fruit. This natural fiber slows down the digestion of fruit so the sugar is released slowly, for slow and steady energy. On the other hand, when you drink fruit juice, the sugar is absorbed quickly (similar to when you eat candy or other simple carbohydrates). This quick rise in your blood sugar can lead to unhealthy energy swings and can send unhealthy messages to your cells.

So instead of drinking soda, sports drinks, or juice, a better choice is just to drink water! Water is the drink that our Earth created for us, to help our bodies function at their best! When you drink water, your brain, your belly, and your body will thank you!

Tip: If you're craving flavor, try adding slices of fruit (like lemon, orange, or cucumber) to your water for a delicious and refreshing twist!

The Problem With Kids' Menus

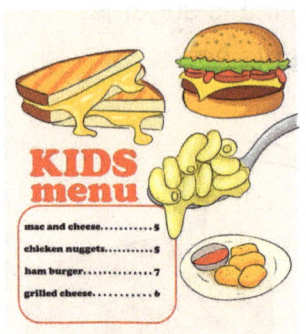

Have you ever noticed that a lot of the kids' menus at most restaurants look kind of similar? They often only have options like mac and cheese, hamburgers, grilled cheese sandwiches, and chicken nuggets, without a lot of options for fruits and vegetables. Also, many of the options don't contain healthy proteins or healthy fats. Not only that, but most of these options are ultra-processed foods— not whole foods.

Why are most kids' menus like this? Well, as we have talked about, many adults have never learned about food and nutrition! They may think that food is all about calories and being healthy is all about how much someone weighs. (After everything we have learned, we know this isn't true!) They also may think that since kids are generally healthy, it's ok for kids to eat mostly ultra-processed foods. But sadly, when kids eat these types of ultra-processed meals, it is not helping their bodies function at their best!

Perhaps the next time you go to a restaurant, or even eat lunch at school, can you look to see if there are any whole foods you can choose? Are there any options where you can eat half fruits and vegetables as part of your plate? Can you pick a meal with healthy proteins and healthy fats and lots of micronutrients?

Now that we've learned how to create a plate filled with delicious, whole foods that nourish our bodies— there's one more extraordinary part of the story.

Have you ever wondered where your food comes from before it ends up on your plate?

The truth is, the power of food doesn't just come from what's on your plate—it begins long before that, on the farms and in the soil, where our food is grown and raised.

To truly understand how incredible food is, we also have to explore the amazing places it begins.

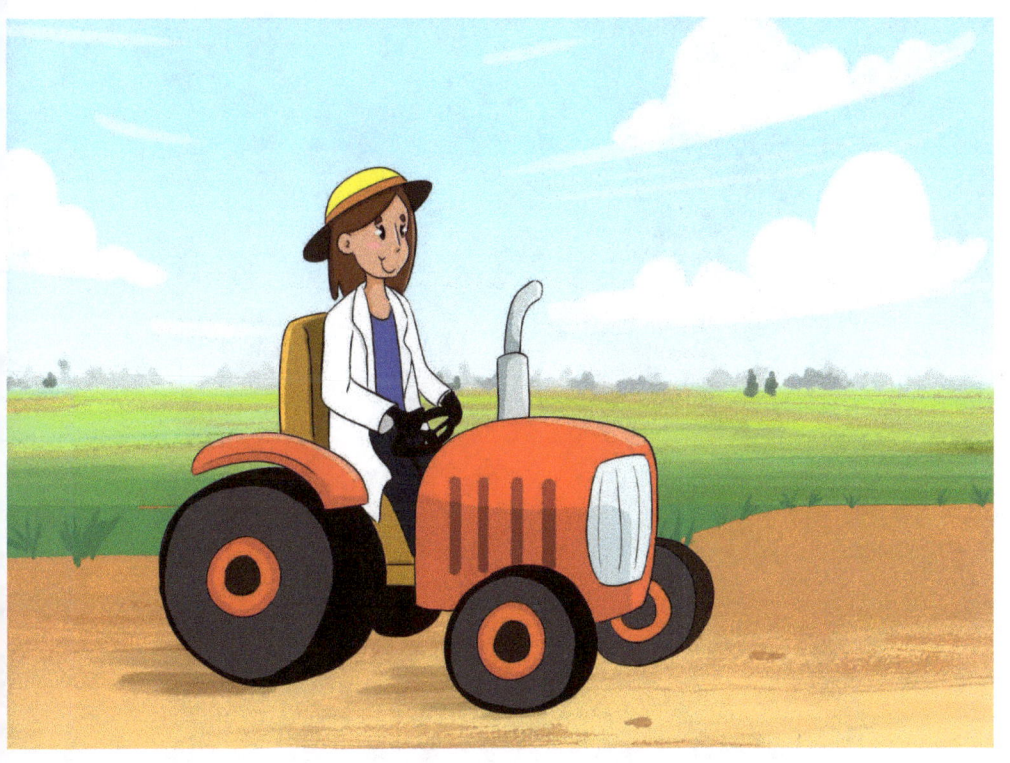

PART 4:
THE CONNECTION BETWEEN OUR BODIES, OUR FOOD, AND OUR EARTH IS **EXTRAORDINARY**

CHAPTER 9
OUR FOOD AND OUR FARMS

Throughout this entire book we have learned that our food is extraordinary! But what if that is just partially true? How does our food become extraordinary?

Do you know where your food was before it reached your plate? Where was your food before it was in your kitchen? Where was your food before it was in the grocery store? How much do you know about the farms where your food was grown?

In order to truly understand the extraordinary power of food we cannot just focus on the food itself. We also need to look at where our food is coming from. When we look closely and start digging deeper, we will see that it may be the farms, the soil, and the air— the Earth where the food is grown that truly make our food incredible!

To understand why this is important, let's start by exploring a little bit about farming methods.

Have you ever heard the terms <u>conventional farming</u> or <u>organic farming</u>? What exactly are they, and what is the difference?

Conventional Farming Practices

The word "conventional" means normal, or what is ordinarily done. Most farms in the United States are conventional farms. Conventional farms use synthetic (human-made) chemical fertilizers to provide nutrients to plants. They also use synthetic pesticides (chemicals to kill pests) and synthetic herbicides (chemicals to kills weeds). These conventional farming methods make it easier for farmers to grow plants faster and increase the amount of crops they can produce.

Conventional farms also often produce <u>GMOs</u> (genetically modified organisms). These are crops where scientists have changed the plant's DNA in a lab to help the plant grow more easily. Many GMO crops have been created to help the crops grow even if they are sprayed with toxic pesticides and herbicides.

Conventional farms also mostly practice mono-cropping. This means that most conventional farms only produce one or a couple types of crops, and the same crops are planted on the same land, year after year.

For example, in the U.S., corn is the most planted crop, and for many farms, it is the only crop that is being produced. For many animal farms in the U.S., they raise only one type of animal.

Conventional farming techniques are considered to be modern techniques because farmers use high tech tools and advanced technologies to increase the amount of food the farmers can grow. But these methods and chemicals cause damage to the soil and the living organisms in the soil. 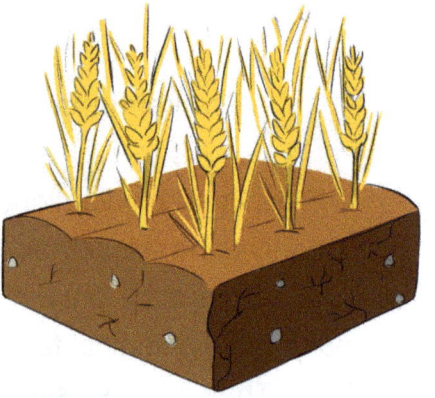 When the soil is damaged and depleted by these methods, it puts these farms at greater risk for problems in the future.

The result? Conventional farms often need to use more and more synthetic fertilizers, pesticides, and herbicides every year, in order for them to be able to produce the same amount of crops.

Organic Farming Practices

Organic farms are different. They mostly rely on natural methods that have been used for thousands of years to keep farms healthy.

Prior to the invention of conventional farming techniques, most farms both grew crops and raised livestock. On these old-fashioned farms, the animals grazed on plants, then deposited manure, which in turn provided nutrients for the crops. This natural system significantly reduced or eliminated the need for additional fertilizers. Most organic farms use these same old-fashioned methods.

Organic farms do not use synthetic chemical pesticides, herbicides, or fertilizers. Instead of synthetic chemical fertilizers, they use natural fertilizers like compost or manure from grazing animals to give nutrients to the soil and plants. These natural fertilizers keep the soil and living organisms in the soil healthy.

Instead of herbicides to kill weeds, organic farms use other plants called "cover crops" to prevent weeds from growing. These cover crops also keep the soil healthy by increasing the nutrients in the soil and reducing pests.

Instead of chemical pesticides, organic farms use more natural substances and other natural methods such as using crop rotation (alternating growing different crops on the same land) to control pests. Crop rotation helps to keep the soil healthy, helps to conserve water, and helps

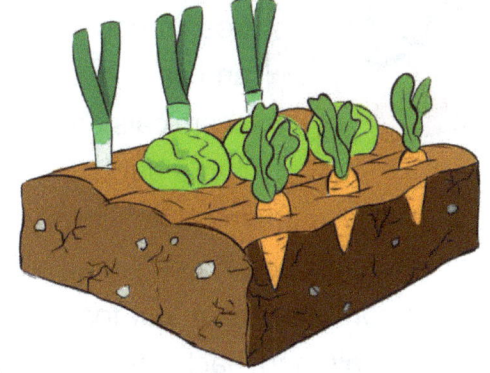

to increase the amount of food that can be harvested. Organic farms also do not grow genetically modified organisms.

Because of all of these differences, conventional and organic farms have different consequences on the health of our Earth and on the health of humans. Let's explore a few of the reasons why.

Pesticides

Did you know that more than 5 billion pounds of pesticides are used worldwide per year? Did you know that many of these pesticides used are in the U.S.? Over a billion pounds of pesticides are used in the U.S. each year to control weeds and insects.

The synthetic chemical fertilizers, synthetic chemical pesticides, and synthetic chemical herbicides used in conventional farms are unhealthy for humans. Many of these chemicals have been found in our food and our water and can cause health problems. These chemicals can even hurt our microbiome in our gut.

These chemical fertilizers, chemical pesticides, and chemical herbicides are also unhealthy for the Earth. In addition to being on our food, they are also washed off with the rain and leach into our soil and pollute our water, causing harm to plants and animals.

Did you know that similar to your microbiome in your body that keeps you healthy, the Earth's soil has a microbiome too? These microbes in the soil keep the soil healthy and full of nutrients. Chemical fertilizers, pesticides, and herbicides damage and kill these microbes too.

On the other hand, organic farms don't use these chemicals, and instead use natural methods to farm. These organic methods don't use unhealthy chemicals for humans, or unhealthy chemicals for plants, animals, or the microbes in the soil. This is just one reason why organic farms are healthier for both humans and the planet.

Antibiotics

Another reason why organic farms are healthier for both humans and the Earth is because conventional animal farms, sometimes called "factory farms," often use antibiotics. Antibiotics are strong medicines used to treat infections by bacteria. Have you ever taken antibiotics to treat a bacterial infection? You may have taken antibiotics in the past if you had an infection on 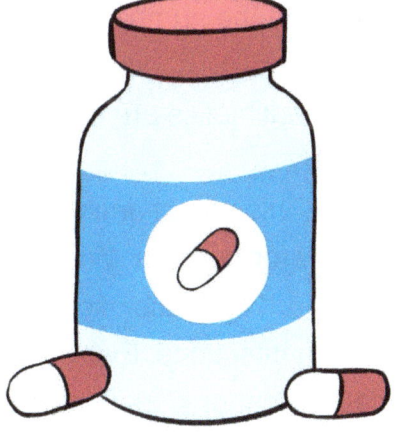 your skin or an infection in your ear. Antibiotics are important medications used by humans to kill harmful bacteria.

(Antibiotics don't kill viruses like cold viruses, flu viruses, or the COVID virus).

While taking antibiotics is super important when needed, it is unhealthy to take antibiotics unnecessarily because they can hurt the microbiome in your body. This is why it is important to only take antibiotics when they are prescribed by a doctor to treat a bacterial infection.

But did you know that 80% of all antibiotics in the United States are sold for use on animal farms? Most of these antibiotics are "medically important," meaning that they are similar to the antibiotics used in human medicine. Unfortunately, though, most of these antibiotics are not being used to actually help animals with infections. Instead, many conventionally farmed animals in the U.S. receive regular low levels of antibiotics in their feed or water- just in case. This way lots of animals can be held together in a very small space, so that the farmers can maximize the number of animals on their farm. These crowded living conditions are unhealthy for the animals, so the antibiotics are used to help prevent disease outbreaks.

This use of antibiotics in conventional farms is not healthy for humans. When these important medicines are overused, the antibiotics can become less effective for fighting infections. Eventually some of these antibiotics may no longer work for humans when we need them. Not only that, but these methods of using antibiotics so that farmers can maximize the number of animals on their farm is unhealthy for the animals and the Earth. Conventional animal farms pollute our water, pollute our air, and pollute the soil.

On the other hand, organic animal farms do not use antibiotics for their animals. This is one reason why, when choosing meat and dairy products, it is best to choose organic products. But not only that, choosing organic "pasture-raised" meat and dairy products is even better. When animals are raised using organic, "pasture-raised" methods, not only are these animals raised without antibiotics, but these animals are also raised in more healthy living conditions. Organic "pasture-raised" animals can go outside and eat grass, rather than spending their entire lives cramped inside a small space with other animals in unhealthy conditions. These organic pasture-raised methods are healthier for the animals and healthier for the Earth. But do you know what is even more amazing? When the animals are raised with these organic pasture-raised methods, the meat, eggs, and dairy products are healthier for humans too!

This is yet another example of why when we farm the way nature and our planet intended us to farm, using organic methods, it is healthier for humans and healthier for the Earth.

Carbon

A third reason why organic farms are healthier for both humans and the Earth is because of carbon! All living things are made of carbon— all plants, all animals, and even you! All living things on this planet are part of our Earth's natural carbon cycle. In this cycle, plants take CO_2 (carbon dioxide) from the air and use that carbon to grow, while they release oxygen in the air. This oxygen in the air is used for animals (including humans) to breathe. Animals breathe in oxygen and then breathe out carbon dioxide into the air. This natural cycle of carbon dioxide and oxygen has stayed balanced for a long time and allows plants and animals to live.

When leaves, plants, and animals die, carbon naturally gets deposited in the earth's soil. Over time, with a lot of heat and pressure, this carbon turns into oil, natural gas and coal that are buried deep underground. Humans discovered that when we dig up this oil, natural gas, and coal, we can use them as fuel to power our cars and homes. These fuels are called "fossil fuels" because they are made from the remains of plants and animals that lived millions of years ago, like the dinosaurs!
While burning these fuels gives humans energy to use, this process also releases extra carbon dioxide into the air. This extra carbon dioxide along with other "greenhouse gases" in the air trap extra heat close to the Earth's surface and can negatively affect the Earth's climate.

THE CARBON CYCLE

CO_2 carbon dioxide

Burning fossil fuels releases extra carbon dioxide into the air.

Plants take carbon dioxide from the air and use that carbon to grow.

This oxygen in the air is used for animals (including humans) to breathe.

Plants release oxygen (O_2) in the air

Animals breathe in oxygen and then breathe out carbon dioxide into the air.

When we dig up these fossil fuels (oil, natural gas, and coal), we can use them as fuel to power our cars and homes.

When leaves, plants, and animals die, carbon naturally gets deposited in the earth's soil.

Over time, with a lot of heat and pressure, this carbon turns into oil, natural gas and coal that are buried deep underground.

fossils and fossil fuel

Conventional farming methods require more energy, use more fossil fuels, and produce more greenhouse gases. For these reasons, conventional farming methods are contributing to the Earth's climate change problem. But not only that, the unhealthy soil on conventional farms, damaged and depleted by synthetic chemicals, also contributes to the problem! Believe it or not, healthy soil can actually act like a sponge and pull carbon dioxide out of the air and trap the carbon back in the Earth's soil. Unfortunately, conventional farming methods that damage the soil prevent the soil from being able to pull and trap the carbon.

On the other hand, organic farming methods, which naturally keep the soil healthy can actually help with the earth's climate change problem! Not only do organic farming methods require less energy and less fossil fuels, but the healthy soil can actually pull carbon dioxide from the atmosphere. This process of carbon trapping helps to deposit the extra carbon back into the Earth's soil, where it belongs. Some scientists have even estimated that if all of the Earth's croplands and pastures were farmed using organic methods that prioritize soil health (called "regenerative organic farming"), it may be possible to soak up all the extra carbon dioxide released by the burning of fossil fuels from an entire year! With less carbon dioxide in the air, the Earth will be healthier, and humans will be healthier too!

CONVENTIONAL FARMING

Traditional farming depletes the soil and releases more carbon into the atmosphere.

ORGANIC FARMING

Regenerative organic agriculture prioritizes soil health. Healthy plants and healthy soil pull more carbon out of the atmosphere.

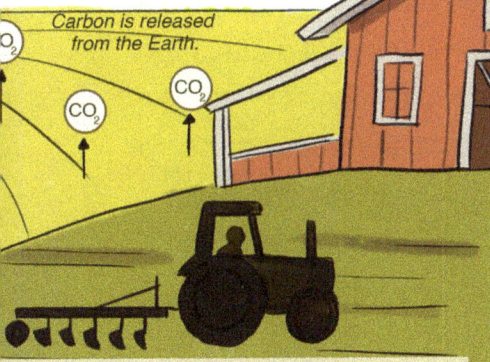

Conventional farming methods (like tilling and using chemical fertilizers and pesticides) use more energy and fossil fuels. They also damage the soil and the microorganisms in the soil. This prevents the soil from being able to pull and trap carbon.

Organic farming methods, which naturally keep the soil healthy require less energy and less fossil fuels. The healthy soil can actually pull carbon dioxide from the atmosphere. This process of carbon trapping helps to deposit the extra carbon back into the Earth's soil, where it belongs.

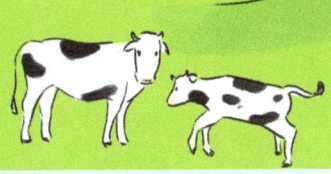

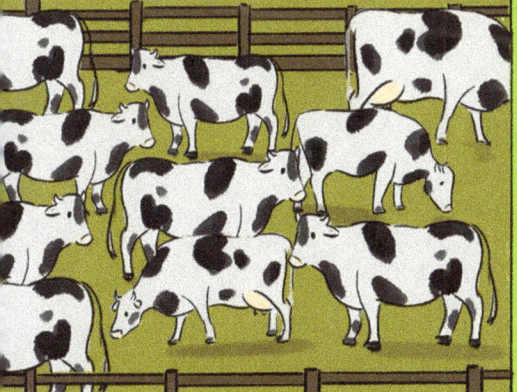

Animals on conventional farms, also called "factory farms," are often held together in a small space. The crowded living conditions can make the animals sick, so antibiotics are often used to prevent disease outbreaks. These methods are unhealthy for the animals, for the Earth and for humans.

When animals are raised using **Organic, Pasture raised** methods, they can go outside and eat grass, and they are raised without antibiotics. This is healthier for the animals and healthier for the Earth. The meat, eggs, and dairy products are healthier for humans too!

So, bottom line, if we farmed the way nature intended us to farm, we would have healthier soil, we would have a healthier planet, we would have healthier food and water, and humans would be healthier too. The connection between our Earth, our food, and our bodies is incredible!

The way we grow our food matters—a lot. It matters for our soil. It matters for our animals. It matters for our water, our air, our climate—and it matters for us.

But here's something even more amazing: It's not just our farming practices that connects our Earth, our food and our bodies. Our food choices connect us too! The same food choices that help keep our bodies strong can also help protect our Earth.

In the next chapter, let's bring it all together—and discover how what's on your plate can shape the future of your health and the future of our planet.

The Cost of Organic Foods

Unfortunately, buying organic foods at the grocery store costs more than buying foods grown with conventional farming. This is because the conventional methods of farming are less expensive than the natural organic methods. This is also because the cost of corn, which is used to make lots of ultra-processed food, and to feed animals on conventional factory farms is low and regulated by the U.S. government.

Since most people don't have extra money to spend, how can families afford to buy organic foods? The good news is that when we buy more plants (fruits, vegetables, beans, lentils, whole grains, nuts, and seeds) and less animal products (steak, pork, chicken, dairy products), we can actually spend less money on our grocery bill! This is especially true if we choose to eat at least a couple meals of plant-based proteins (ex. beans, lentils, or tofu) instead of meat.

For example, the cost of steak is about $10-20 dollars per pound. On the other hand, the cost of 1 pound of organic black beans is less than $2 dollars per pound. Then, after you cook the pound of black beans, it will turn into more than 6 pounds of organic black beans. With that in mind, steak is about 45 times more expensive than organic black beans!

The Cost of Organic Food and Saving Money By Eating More Plants

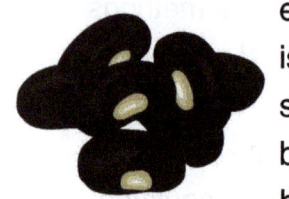

Not only are black beans much more affordable but eating black beans as a source of protein is also healthier for your body than eating steak (red meat). Plant based proteins like beans, lentils, tofu, nuts, and seeds all have lots of fiber, lots of micronutrients, and are all great choices!

Even if you can substitute a few meals a week of eating less meat and more plant-based proteins like beans, lentils, or tofu instead, your family will save a lot of money! This saved money can be used to choose organic foods!

CHAPTER 10
OUR INCREDIBLE FOOD, OUR INCREDIBLE BODIES, OUR INCREDIBLE EARTH

Everything we've learned so far—about food, our bodies, our microbiome, our genes, and our farms—comes together in one extraordinary truth:

The health of our bodies and the health of our Earth are deeply connected.

Just like your body needs nutrients to grow and thrive, the Earth needs care and nourishment too. And guess what? When we choose to eat more whole foods—especially plants—we're not just helping ourselves… we're also helping our planet.

So, in this chapter, let's take a look at how every bite we take can shape a healthier future—for us and for the world we share.

Let's review what we have learned about whole foods. When we eat more whole foods, the foods that the Earth created for us, it will help our bodies function at their best.

First, we learned that when we eat whole food sources of carbohydrates, including fruits, vegetables, beans, lentils, and whole grains, we are eating mostly complex carbohydrates that give us lasting sustained energy! This will help us feel less tired and more energetic!

Second, we learned that when we eat whole food sources of protein, including fish, lean meats, eggs, beans, lentils, tofu, nuts, and seeds we help our muscles get stronger.

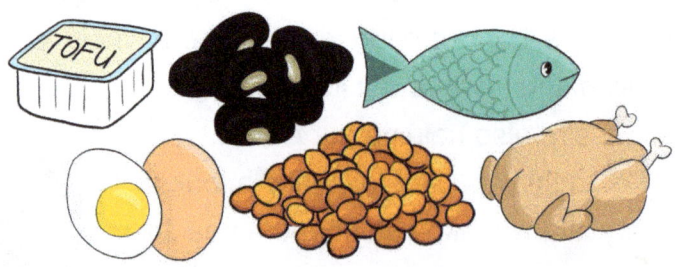

Third, we learned that when we eat healthy fats including nuts, nut butters, seeds, avocados, olives, and fish, we help our brain get stronger and sharper!

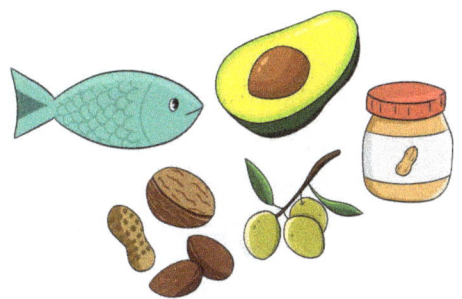

Fourth, we learned that when we eat lots of whole foods, including fruits and vegetables, we will be eating food with loads of micronutrients and phytonutrients. These micronutrients help our body thrive!

Fifth, we learned that when we eat plant sources of whole foods, including fruits, vegetables, beans, lentils, whole grains, nuts, and seeds, we will be eating lots of fiber, which helps nourish our microbiome to be healthier and happier, which will in turn help us feel healthier and happier.

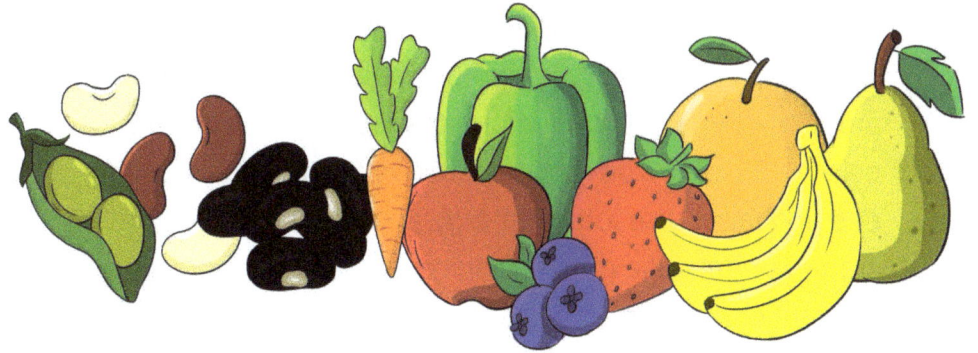

Lastly, we learned that when we eat whole foods, we will be sending good messages to our genes and our cells, which help us influence our genes and cells in a positive way and stay healthy in the future!

Eating mostly whole foods is the best way to help our bodies feel good now and to create a healthy future!

But eating mostly whole foods also helps the Earth! Let's explore why.

Since whole foods are foods found in nature, they don't require as much energy to produce as ultra-processed foods, which are made in big factories. Whole foods also usually come with less packaging, which means less plastic waste. Additionally, when we eat whole foods, it is also possible to choose organic whole foods that are grown locally. Eating organic foods keeps the soil healthy and reduces pollution. Eating food that is grown locally reduces the distance that food needs to be shipped and can also help reduce pollution.

On the other hand, ultra-processed foods—like packaged snacks, sugary cereals, fast food, and soda—are created in big factories and the ingredients typically come from large conventional factory farms. These factories and farms use lots of energy and fossil fuels, which create greenhouse gas emissions. As we learned, the conventional farms also use methods that harm the soil, pollute water, and damage the planet's ecosystems.

Ultra-processed foods also typically come in plastic packages which contribute to pollution and waste disposal issues. Not only that, but ultra-processed foods are typically shipped long distances, which burns even more fossil fuels and contributes to climate change.

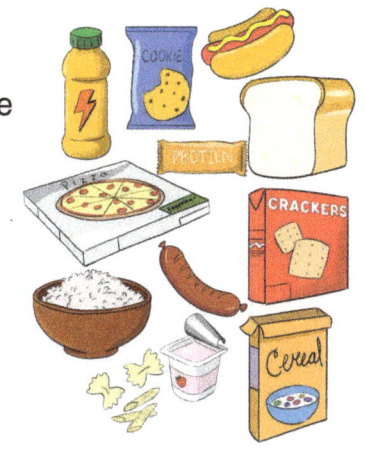

So, every time we choose whole foods over ultra-processed ones, we're making a powerful choice to protect our bodies and to protect our planet.

And guess what? Choosing to eat more plants is also healthier for humans and healthier for the Earth!

We have already learned why eating lots of plants is healthy for your body. When you eat lots of plants (fruits, vegetables, beans, lentils, nuts, seeds, and whole grains), you get lots of fiber, healthy fats, lots of micronutrients, and lots of phytonutrients, which all help your body thrive! This is why you want to make sure that for every meal, half of your plate is fruits and vegetables. This is also why you want to include foods like beans, lentils, nuts, seeds, and tofu on your plate as sources of healthy protein.

When you eat more plants, you will automatically have less room on your plate for meat and dairy products. This also helps the Earth! Let's explore why.

Growing plants takes a lot less energy, water, and

land than raising animals for meat and dairy. Many conventional farms grow huge amounts of corn just to feed farm animals like cows, chickens, and pigs. But here's the problem—these animals eat way more food than they give back to us as meat or milk. That means a lot of food is used up just to feed them!

If everyone on Earth ate more plants, and even a little less meat and dairy products, this would help make sure that more people around the world can have enough healthy food to eat.

Raising farm animals for meat and dairy also creates more pollution than growing plants. When we eat more plants and fewer animals, farms will use less energy, water, and land, and they will produce less pollution. When we eat more plant foods, we also leave more land and resources for farmers to use organic and sustainable farming methods that are better for the animals and better for the planet.

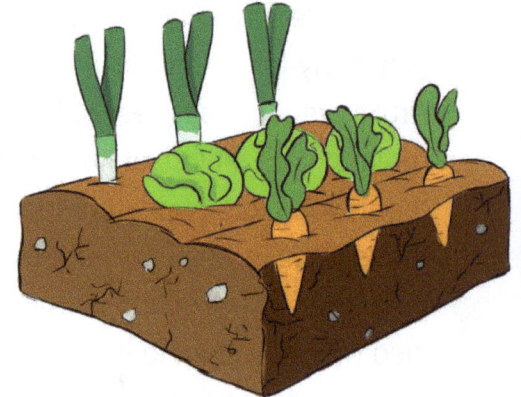

So, if we all eat even just a little less meat and dairy, while we also eat more plants, the farmers could use better, organic methods, the Earth would be healthier (less pollution, better farming), and humans would be healthier too!

Our Earth is extraordinary! The food which the Earth has created for us is extraordinary! And you—your body, your mind, your heart—are extraordinary too.

In 1974, Sir Albert Howard, a scientist who is one of the founders of organic farming said, "The health of soil, plant, animal and man is one and indivisible." With all of our scientific advances, more and more, we are learning that this could not be more true.

Everything is connected. The health of our soil, the plants that grow from it, the food we eat, the way we feel, how we grow, how we live, and the health of our planet—it's all part of one beautiful, interconnected system.

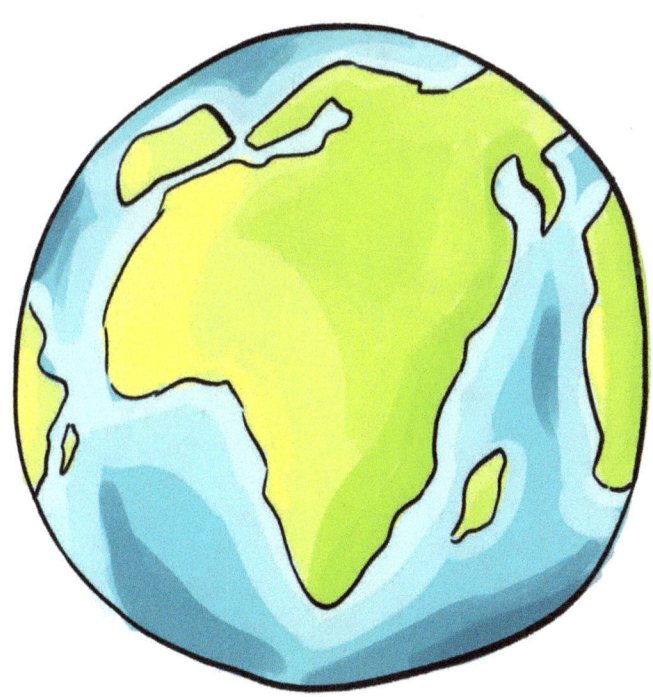

So now that you know the truth, what will you choose? Will you choose foods that help your body feel energized, focused, and strong? Will you choose foods that help your microbiome thrive and your brain feel calm and happy? Will you choose foods that send good messages to your genes, so you stay healthy for years to come? Will you choose foods that protect our Earth, our animals, our soil, our water, and our future?

You don't have to be perfect. But every time you eat, you have a chance to make a powerful choice.

You have the power to take care of your body.
You have the power to take care of our Earth.
That power begins with what you put on your plate.

Set a Goal to Help Your Body and the Earth!

Now that you have learned how the food you eat can help your brain, your body, your microbiome, and even the planet, it's your turn to take action!

Set a goal for yourself this week. Start small—but think big!

☑ Want to help your brain?
Goal idea: I will eat one food with healthy fats (like nuts or avocado) every day.

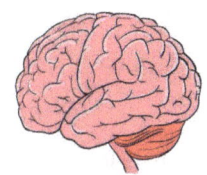

☑ Want to help your microbiome?
Goal idea: I will eat six fruits or veggies with fiber every day.

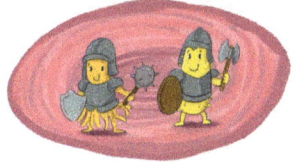

☑ Want to help the Earth?
Goal idea: I will eat two plant-based meals this week instead of meat.

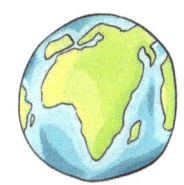

☑ Want to feel more energy?
Goal idea: I will drink water instead of soda or juice five times this week.

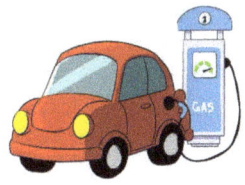

Every healthy choice you make helps your body AND our planet. Even small changes can add up to big results! You are making a difference!

Be The Teacher At Home

Do you think that the connection between our food, our bodies, and our Earth is extraordinary? Do you wish that everyone knew this information, so that you, your family, your friends, and our Earth could be healthier?

If so, tell your family and friends about what you have learned! Read this book together with your parents. You might even inspire your family to try a new food or make a healthy change together!

Sharing what you've learned will help the people you love feel healthier! And when more people understand the power of food, it will help our Earth too!

What is one thing you want to tell others about the power of food?

AFTERWORD:

When I was growing up, no one ever told me how powerful food could be.

I didn't know that what I ate could change how I felt. I didn't know that my food choices could protect my body— or protect the planet. I had to learn these things as an adult. And honestly, I wish I had known them much earlier.

This is why I wrote this book.

Because I believe you—and every kid—deserve to know the truth. You deserve to know how amazing your body is. You deserve to know how much your choices matter. And I hope, more than anything, that this book helps you feel inspired to make choices that help you feel your best— strong, smart, energized, and proud— for the rest of your life!

The food you eat matters. **You** matter. And our world is better when you understand the wonder of what we eat.

With love and belief in your power,

Dr. Ritu Saluja-Sharma

GLOSSARY:

Anthocyanins (an-tho-SY-uh-ninz): Natural pigments that give red, purple, and blue colors to fruits and vegetables.

Aspartame (AS-par-tame): An artificial sweetener often used in diet sodas and sugar-free gum.

Bran (BRAN): The outer layer of whole grains, which is full of fiber and nutrients.

Carbohydrates (kar-bo-HY-drayts): Nutrients that give your body energy, found in foods like fruits and vegetables, grains, beans, and lentils.

Carotenoids (ka-ROT-uh-noyds): Natural pigments in plants that give yellow, orange, and red colors, like in carrots.

Cells (SELZ): The tiny building blocks that make up every part of your body.

Chyme (KYM): A thick, soupy mix of food and stomach juices that helps with digestion.

Complex Carbohydrates (KOM-pleks kar-bo-HY-drayts): Long chains of simple sugars linked together, which take your body time to break down. Examples are foods like whole grains, beans, and vegetables, which give long-lasting energy.

Conventional (kun-VEN-shuh-nul) Farming: A way of growing food using regular farming methods, using human-made chemicals.

Corn Starch (KORN STARCH): A powder made from corn that thickens sauces and soups.

Cobalamin (co-BAL-uh-min): Also known as Vitamin B12, helps keep your blood and nerve cells healthy.

Cruciferous Vegetables (kroo-SIF-er-uhs VEJ-tuh-buhlz): A group of powerful veggies like broccoli, cabbage, and kale that are very healthy.

Dextrose (DEKS-trohs): A type of sugar made from corn, used to sweeten food.

Dopamine (DOH-puh-meen): A brain chemical that helps you feel happy and motivated.

Edamame (ed-uh-MAH-may): Green soybeans that are often boiled and eaten as a snack.

Endosperm (EN-doh-sperm): The starchy center part of a grain that is separated from the other parts of the grain and used in refined grains, like white bread and white rice.

Enzymes (EN-zymz): Special proteins that help speed up chemical reactions in your body.

Epigenetics (ep-i-jeh-NET-iks): The study of how your genes can change based on your environment and habits.

Erythritol (eh-RITH-rih-tol): An artificial sweetener often used in sugar-free foods.

Fat (FAT): A nutrient found in foods like oil, butter, avocados, nuts, and seeds, that gives energy, helps your body absorb vitamins, and is important for the structure of cells.

Fiber (FY-bur): A part of plants that your body can't digest, but helps keep your microbiome and digestive tract healthy.

GABA (GAB-uh): (Stands for Gamma-Aminobutyric Acid) A chemical messenger in your brain that helps you feel calm and relaxed.

Germ (JERM): The tiny part of a grain seed that has nutrients to help the plant grow.

Glucose (GLOO-kohs): A simple sugar that your body uses for energy.

GMO (G-M-O): A genetically modified organism, where scientists change a plant or animal's DNA.

High Fructose Corn Syrup (high FROOK-tohs KORN sir-up): A sweet liquid made from corn that's often used to flavor ultra-processed foods.

Macronutrients (mak-ro-NOO-tree-uhnts): Nutrients your body needs in large amounts, like carbohydrates, protein, and fat.

Magnesium (mag-NEE-zee-um): An important mineral found in beans, seeds, nuts, and green leafy vegetables that helps muscles work and keeps your heart healthy.

Mannitol (MAN-ih-tol): An artificial sweetener found in some processed foods.

Microbe (MY-kroh-b): A tiny living thing, like bacteria.

Microbiome (MY-kroh-BY-ohm): The community of tiny living things that live in your body, especially your digestive tract (your gut microbiome).

Micronutrients (MY-kroh-NOO-tree-uhnts): Vitamins and minerals that your body needs in order to function properly.

Myofibrils (MY-oh-FY-brils): Tiny fibers in muscles made mostly of protein, that help them contract and move.

Neurotransmitters (NOO-roh-trans-MIT-urz): Chemicals in your brain that send messages between nerve cells.

Omega 3 Fats (oh-MAY-guh three fats): Healthy fats found in fish, nuts, and seeds that help your brain and heart.

Organic (or-GAN-ik) Farming: Food grown without human-made chemicals or GMOs (genetically modified organisms).

Phytonutrients (FYE-toh-NOO-tree-uhnts): Natural chemicals found in plants that help keep your body healthy.

Polyunsaturated Fat (PAH-lee-un-SAT-uh-ray-ted fat): A type of fat found in some oils, fish, nuts, and seeds. Omega 3 fatty acids and Omega 6 fatty acids are types of polyunsaturated fat.

Protein (PRO-teen): An important nutrient that builds muscles and repairs your body.

Quinoa (KEEN-wah): A type of healthy whole grain, that's high in protein, and is prepared in a similar way to rice.

Riboflavin (RYE-bo-flay-vin): Also known as Vitamin B2, helps turn food into energy.

Saccharin (SAK-uh-rin): An artificial sweetener that is often used in soft drinks and "diet" products.

Salmonella (sal-muh-NEL-uh): A harmful bacteria that can cause food poisoning, often from undercooked meat or eggs.

Serotonin (ser-oh-TOH-nin): A chemical in your brain that helps you feel happy and calm.

Simple Carbohydrates (SIM-puhl kar-bo-HY-drayts): A food made of simple sugars that break down quickly in your body, like candy or white bread.

Sorbitol (SOR-bih-tol): An artificial sweetener used in sugar-free candies and gums.

Sucralose (SOO-kruh-lohs): An artificial sweetener that tastes like sugar and is used in baked goods and drinks.

Sulforaphane (sul-FOR-uh-fane): A natural plant nutrient (phytonutrient) found in cruciferous vegetables (like broccoli, kale, and cauliflower) that is super powerful, and helps with heart health, brain health, and the health of your cells.

Thiamine (THY-uh-meen): Also known as Vitamin B1, helps your body turn food into energy.

Whole Grain (HOHL grayn): Grains that include all parts of the seed, like bran, germ, and endosperm. Examples are brown rice, 100% whole wheat bread, and quinoa, that are healthier than refined grains (white bread, white rice).

Xanthan Gum (ZAN-than gum): A thickener made from corn, used in food to give it texture.

Xylitol (ZY-lih-tol): An artificial sweetener that is often used in sugar-free gums and candy.

ABOUT THE AUTHOR

Dr. Ritu Saluja-Sharma, MD, is a double board-certified physician in Emergency Medicine and Lifestyle Medicine, and the founder of Head Heart Hands—a comprehensive, holistic wellness program for individuals and organizations. She is also a devoted mother and a passionate advocate for food-based health education.

After years of practicing Emergency Medicine on the frontlines of our healthcare system and seeing many of her patients suffering with diseases that could likely have been prevented, (and many which could potentially still be reversed), Dr. Saluja-Sharma created Head Heart Hands to help people prevent and reverse disease by targeting ROOT CAUSES.

While searching for ways to make her programs accessible to all, she expanded from individual coaching to working with corporations and school systems, offering her online and corporate programs to people of all demographics and education levels, to help people lower their blood sugars, blood pressure, and cholesterol, increase their energy, improve their mood, decrease their pain, and improve their quality of life.

After witnessing incredible transformations in adults, she turned her attention to children—knowing that the earlier healthy habits are formed, the more lasting they can be.

Through her book and companion workbook, she's empowering a new generation to understand the power of food, build healthy mindsets, and fall in love with their bodies and the nourishment that fuels them. She is currently working to improve the health and nutrition curriculum in public schools and serves as an expert advisor on state-level curriculum standards.

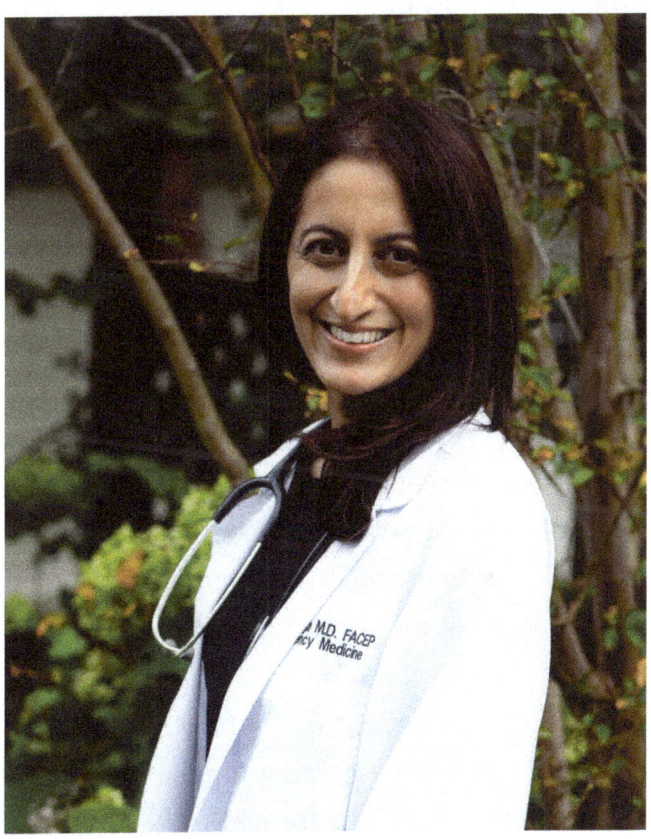

ACKNOWLEDGMENTS

This book would not exist without the support, inspiration, and encouragement of so many wonderful people.

To my husband—my one and only Board of Director—thank you for always being there, for your thoughtful advice (no matter how often I ask), and for your unwavering support through every stage of this project.

To my incredible children—you were the first to read this book and were always so kind, encouraging, and proud of your mommy. Your support and enthusiasm meant the world to me. You've not only inspired this project, but also became my co-authors for the companion workbook and cookbook. It was while preparing to speak in your classroom—and realizing how few children's books talk about food and nutrition in the way I believe matters—that I saw how much this book was needed. Your curiosity, honesty, and joyful spirit fuel my passion to help other children learn, grow, and thrive too.

To my parents and sister, thank you for always cheering me on, lending a hand, and offering encouragement in all the ways that matter most.

To all my friends at Montgomery County Public Schools (MCPS) and Frederick County Public Schools (FCPS)—your excitement and support helped give this book its wings. Thank you for believing in the vision and for helping me bring it to life in the classroom and beyond.

To the Pritcher family, thank you for being the very first to read the manuscript. Your feedback, kind words, and early encouragement gave me the boost I needed to keep going.

To Navdeep, thank you for sharing your incredible talent with such kindness and care. You've been an absolute joy to work with.

Each of you has played a part in making this book what it is. I am deeply grateful.

Keep Learning, Keep Growing!
Loved this book? There's more to explore!

The Wonder of What We Eat is just the beginning. Keep the journey going with these two exciting companions:

The Wonder of What We Eat Workbook

Turn everything you've learned into action!
Packed with fun activities, reflection prompts, label reading, and real-world challenges, the workbook helps kids apply what they learned to build confidence, make healthy choices, and develop lifelong habits.

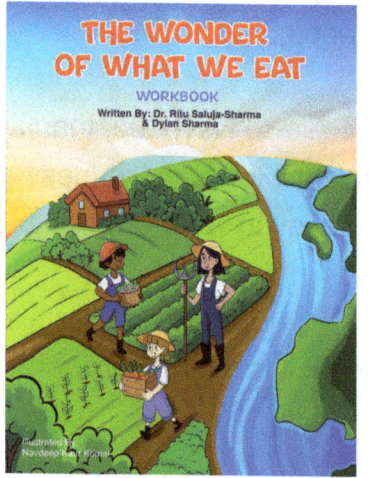

Whether used at home, in classrooms, or with health professionals, this workbook is already making an impact. Lessons are currently being used in one of the largest public school systems in the country—bringing engaging, prevention-focused health education to thousands of students.

Ready to turn knowledge into real-life transformation?
Take the next step—with The Wonder of What We Eat Workbook.

The Wonder of What We Eat Cookbook

Practice everything you have learned in the kitchen to make healthy meals the whole family can enjoy!

Packed with easy, delicious, and nourishing recipes made with real ingredients—designed to support growing bodies, sharp minds, and steady moods.

Make healthy eating fun and doable at home, with kid-approved meals that even picky eaters can get excited about, step-by-step instructions that empower kids to cook on their own or alongside a parent, and built-in learning moments, helping kids understand how food supports their health in ways they can see and feel.

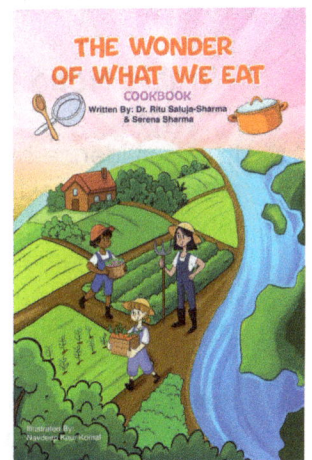

Want to help your kids build lifelong healthy habits, confidence in the kitchen, and a love for real, nourishing food?
Make it happen—with *The Wonder of What We Eat Cookbook*.

Together, the three books form the Head Heart Hands collection:
Book = Head ⟶ Learn the science
Workbook = Heart ⟶ Reflect and apply
Cookbook = Hands ⟶ Take action in the kitchen

Build a healthy relationship with food and your body—for life!

For Grown-Ups Who Want to Feel Better, Too

If this book inspired you to think differently about food and health for your kids, you're not alone. Many adults reading this have asked the same question:
"Where was this information when I was growing up?"

The truth is—it's never too late to start.
Dr. Ritu Saluja-Sharma, the author of *The Wonder of What We Eat*, is also the founder of **Head Heart Hands**.

What is Head Heart Hands?

It's an evidence-based, physician-created, proven, step-by-step program addressing all aspects of health including insulin resistance, inflammation, nutrition, and weight loss, but also stress, sleep, and mental health, designed to help you lose weight, increase your energy, and lower your blood sugars, cholesterol, and blood pressure in 12 Weeks.

Head ⟶ Step-By-Step Guidance and Mindset: Understand the Root Causes of our most common physical and mental health disorders. Learn how to target those root causes to help you lose weight, increase your energy, lower your blood sugars, decrease your cholesterol, and reduce your blood pressure, without medications.

Heart ⟶ Hope and Support: Our bodies are powerful and miraculous and are often capable of healing themselves. Improve your relationship with food, your body, and your health. Ditch dieting and instead focus on nourishment and self-care.

Hands ⟶ Tools and Reach: Implement positive changes into your life by using the many tools from this program, including meal plans, recipes, grocery lists, and challenges. Transcend the confines of hospitals and doctors' offices to meet you where you are- at school, at work, and at home.

Learn More
To explore online adult programs, corporate wellness, and hospital or school system partnerships:
Visit headhearthandsmd.com
Or follow along on Instagram: @head_heart_handsmd

A 12 WEEK JOURNEY OF WELLNESS AND WEIGHT LOSS

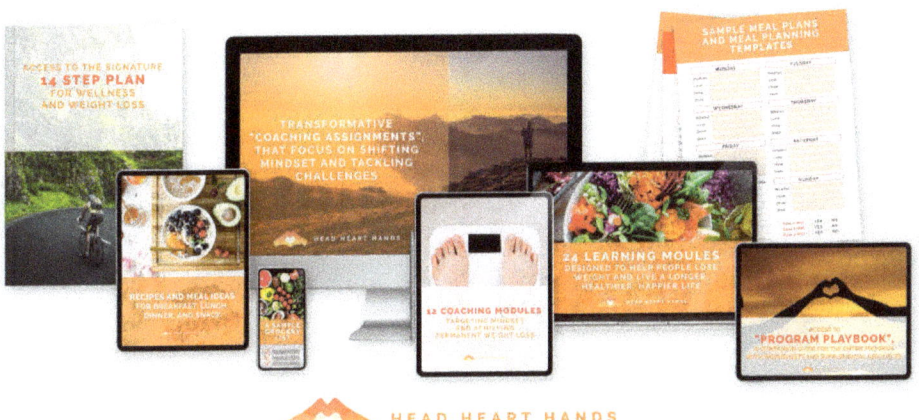

"Everyone wants to live a long and healthy life, free of disease and free of medications. But in order to achieve this, we need the guidance, support, and tools to target the root causes of our problems— so we can prevent and reverse disease. Unfortunately, in our healthcare system, the emphasis is mostly just on disease management and expensive pharmaceuticals, not disease prevention and reversal— leaving most of the patients that I see feeling powerless and frustrated with their health. I understand, because in the past, I have felt that way too.

I believe that everyone should have the right to the guidance, support and tools, to prevent and reverse disease and feel their best— and this is why I created my Head Heart Hands programs, which have empowered so many participants transform their health and transform their life, in just 12 weeks."

-Dr. Ritu Saluja-Sharma

www.ingramcontent.com/pod-product-compliance
Lightning Source LLC
Chambersburg PA
CBHW060948050426
42337CB00052B/1828